To Chris Buckland-Wright

with warmest personal regard

Kns

5 Jun 1987

STUDIES IN OSTEOARTHROSIS
PATHOGENESIS, INTERVENTION, ASSESSMENT

STUDIES IN OSTEOARTHROSIS

PATHOGENESIS, INTERVENTION, ASSESSMENT

EDITED BY

D. J. LOTT, M. K. JASANI and G. F. B. BIRDWOOD

A Wiley Medical Publication

JOHN WILEY & SONS

CHICHESTER • NEW YORK • BRISBANE • TORONTO • SINGAPORE

British Library Cataloguing in Publication Data:

Studies in osteoarthrosis: pathogenesis,
    intervention, assessment.
    1. Osteoarthrosis
    I. Lott, D.J.   II. Jasani, M.K.
    III. Birdwood, G.F.B.
    616.7′2   RC933
    ISBN 0 471 91336 7

Library of Congress Cataloging in Publication Data:

Studies in osteoarthrosis.
    (A Wiley medical publication)
    Includes bibliographies and index.
    1. Osteoarthritis.   I. Lott, D.J.   II. Jasani, M.K.
    III. Birdwood, G.F.B.
    IV. Series. [DNLM: 1. Osteoarthritis. WE 348 S933]
    RC931.067S78   1987   616.7′22   86–23428
    ISBN 0 471 91336 7

Filmset and printed in Great Britain by
BAS Printers Limited, Over Wallop, Hampshire

Contents

EFFECTS OF INTERVENTION ON THE PROCESSES OF OA

Editors and Contributors

M. T. BAYLISS
Experimental Pathology Unit, Institute of Orthopaedics, Royal National Orthopaedic Hospital, Stanmore, Middlesex (now at The Kennedy Institute of Rheumatology, London), UK

G. F. B. BIRDWOOD
Ciba-Geigy Scientific Publications, London, UK

M. C. BUTLER
Research Department, Pharmaceuticals Division, Ciba-Geigy Corporation, Ardsley, New York, USA

J. J. CHART
Research Department, Pharmaceuticals Division, Ciba-Geigy Corporation, Ardsley, New York, USA

C. COLOMBO
Research Department, Pharmaceuticals Division, Ciba-Geigy Corporation, Ardsley, New York, USA

PAUL DIEPPE
University Department of Medicine, Bristol Royal Infirmary, Bristol, UK

D. L. GARDNER
Department of Histopathology, University Hospital of South Manchester, UK

D. M. GRENNAN
University of Manchester Rheumatic Diseases Centre, Hope Hospital, Manchester, UK

F. D. HART
Consultant Rheumatologist, Harley Street, London, formerly Westminster Hospital, London, UK

L. Y. HICKMAN
Research Department, Pharmaceuticals Division, Ciba-Geigy Corporation, Ardsley, New York, USA

E. C. HUSKISSON
St Bartholomew's Hospital, London, UK

M. K. JASANI
Ciba-Geigy Pharmaceuticals, Horsham, UK

M. I. V. JAYSON
Rheumatic Diseases Centre, Hope Hospital, University of Manchester, UK

D. J. LOTT
Ciba-Geigy Pharmaceuticals, Horsham, UK

G. LUST
James A. Baker Institute for Animal Health, New York State College of Veterinary Medicine, Cornell University, Ithaca, New York, USA

R. MAIER
Research Department, Pharmaceuticals Division, Ciba-Geigy Ltd, Basle, Switzerland

R. MAZURYK
Department of Pathology, Medical Academy, Szczecin, Poland

J. NOBLE
University of Manchester, UK

E. M. O'BYRNE
Research and Development Department, Pharmaceuticals Division, Ciba-Geigy Corporation, Ardsley, New York, USA

P. O'CONNOR
Department of Histopathology, University Hospital of South Manchester, UK

J. C. QUINTAVALLA
Research and Development Department, Pharmaceuticals Division, Ciba-Geigy Corporation, Ardsley, New York, USA

H. SCHRODER
Research and Development Department, Pharmaceuticals Division, Ciba-Geigy Corporation, Ardsley, New York, USA

L. SOLOMON
Department of Orthopaedic Surgery, University of the Witwatersrand, Johannesburg, South Africa (now at the University of Bristol Medical School, and Southmead Hospital, Bristol, UK)

B. G. STEINETZ
Research Department, Pharmaceuticals Division, Ciba-Geigy Corporation, Ardsley, New York (now at the Laboratory for Experimental Medicine and Surgery in Primates, New York University Medical Center), USA

C. STRAWINSKI
Research and Development Department, Pharmaceuticals Division, Ciba-Geigy Corporation, Ardsley, New York, USA

D. C. SWARTZENDRUBER
Research Department, Pharmaceuticals Division, Ciba-Geigy Corporation, Ardsley, New York, USA

I. WATT
Department of Radiodiagnosis, Bristol Royal Infirmary, Bristol, UK

G. WILHELMI
Research Department, Pharmaceuticals Division, Ciba-Geigy Ltd, Basle, Switzerland

M. WOODWORTH
Research Department, Pharmaceuticals Division, Ciba-Geigy Corporation, Ardsley, New York, USA

N. B. WURSTER
James A. Baker Institute for Animal Health, New York State College of Veterinary Medicine, Cornell University, Ithaca, New York, USA

Preface

For a common disabling condition, OA gives rise to a surprisingly broad range of questions—from its causation to its possible future prevention or cure—that have yet to be fully resolved. The papers collected here focus on three key areas:

—The nature of the processes that mediate joint damage in OA

—The means for intervening in those processes, prophylactically or therapeutically, and

—The value of the methods available for assessing changes in joint damage, and thus the natural history or the benefits of intervention, whether in individual patients or in clinical trials.

Many questions remain to be answered in each of these problem areas, but we trust that this publication—originally inspired by a workshop meeting on the same topics—will serve both to enlighten the reader and to stimulate future studies.

D. J. Lott

M. K. Jasani

G. F. B. Birdwood

Foreword

The aims of research into the nature and treatment of OA

F. DUDLEY HART

All over the world the most common incapacitating and potentially crippling form of chronic joint disease is osteoarthrosis (OA) of the hip and knee. Pain, stiffness and weakness prevent normal function, leading to loss of mobility, lowered morale and inability to live a normal and fulfilling life. To intervene more effectively we need to learn more about the causation of OA and the mechanisms by which it causes joint damage. The ultimate aim must be to intervene before such damage has occurred, or at least before it has begun to cause pain and disability. The detailed anatomical and biochemical studies reported here show where future progress may be made.

The current drug treatment of OA depends primarily on the non-steroidal anti-inflammatory drugs (NSAIDs) which maintain mobility and function by easing pain and stiffness in the affected tissues, enabling the patient to perform daily tasks more effectively with less discomfort. It was apparent from the early days of phenylbutazone in 1952, and indomethacin 12 years later, that NSAIDs relieve the pain of OA more than the simple analgesics in most, though not all, cases and are generally better tolerated than large doses of aspirin. The inflammatory synovial element in OA also responds to the NSAIDs more effectively than to the simple analgesic agents, such as paracetamol.

There are now sufficient NSAIDs for patients to change from one to another if the clinical response is inadequate or unwanted side effects appear. Although other drugs, including anxiolytics, antidepressants, iron and vitamins, may be indicated on occasion, they are needed less often than in the treatment of rheumatoid arthritis. In a chronic painful disorder like OA, potentially addictive drugs play no part in day-to-day management, and corticosteroids are contraindicated, apart from occasional intra-articular injections in acute inflammatory episodes.

But what of the long-term effects of regular NSAID therapy? Do some or all of these agents, used over prolonged periods, damage the joints they are intended to help? Personally, I have been worried by the development of Charcot-like joints in some patients, during the past 30 years, but impressed by the symptomatic improvement often produced by suitable medication.

The risk/benefit balance has been discussed in the *Journal of Rheumatology* under the title 'NSAIDs and OA—help or hindrance?'. The authors point out that the NSAIDs have significant effects on many of the processes, protective or destructive, concerned in cartilage degeneration. They emphasise the need for systematic study of the relationship between synovial inflammation and cartilage destruction, and of the effects of NSAIDs on each of these processes.

These are major questions, to which the papers published here provide some valuable and, in part, reassuring answers. As clinicians treating patients with OA, we need to know much more about the long-term results of the different forms of treatment we prescribe for this very common and variable disorder.

REFERENCE

BROOKS, P. M., POTTER, S. R. and BUCHANAN, W. W. (1982) NSAIDs and OA—help or hindrance? *J. Rheumatol.* **9**, 3.

PROCESSES
AT WORK
IN OA

Chapter 1

Clinical Aspects of Osteoarthritis

PAUL DIEPPE

University Department of Medicine, Bristol Royal Infirmary, Bristol, UK

NATURE OF THE CONDITION

Osteoarthritis can be defined as a group of synovial joint diseases characterised by loss of the articular cartilage with increased activity of the underlying bone. This simple pathological concept is reflected in the typical radiological changes, which include joint space narrowing (due to cartilage loss), subarticular sclerosis, cysts, and osteophytes (due to increased bone activity). Epidemiological studies and clinical diagnosis are usually based on these radiographic changes, there being no pathognomonic clinical, biochemical or other marker of the disorder.

Clinical surveys of osteoarthritis vary in their emphasis. Some authors have concentrated on patients presenting with monoarticular disease of, for example, the hip (Solomon, 1976), others on post-traumatic changes at a single joint site (Johnson *et al.*, 1974), whereas some papers describe a polyarticular disease affecting both large and small joints (Kellgren and Moore, 1952).

Epidemiological surveys stress the frequency of the disorder, but also indicate that many patients with radiological evidence of advanced disease remain asymptomatic (Lawrence, 1963), and that the disease behaves differently in different joint sites and in different racial groups.

Animal models of osteoarthritis include those in which joint trauma is induced and inbred strains which develop the disease spontaneously. Of necessity, pathological and radiological changes are used to assess the disorder. It is therefore important to establish the degree to which predisposition and post-traumatic changes operate in the human disease, and to examine the relationship between pathology and clinical presentations. This introductory paper briefly examines the heterogeneity of human osteoarthritis, and the causes of symptoms.

HETEROGENEITY OF OSTEOARTHRITIS

It is now clear that osteoarthritis is not a single disease entity. Many authors prefer to regard it as 'joint failure', a process which can result from several different diseases (Ali, 1978).

Osteoarthritis is usually classified according to the presence or absence of any obvious aetiological factor (primary or secondary). It can be divided into monoarticular and polyarticular forms: monoarticular OA is often said to be secondary to some traumatic or mechanical factor; polyarticular OA is often described as primary. However, this distinction may be too simplistic, as illustrated by the work of Doherty *et al.* (1983), and the incidence of polyarticular involvement is a function of how hard one looks for it.

Factors thought to be important in the development of OA include genetics (especially in generalised disease), trauma, age, abnormal joint mechanics, metabolic predisposition, and inflammatory joint disease. A wide variety of different forms of 'joint failure' are seen, behaving entirely differently at different joint sites and in different age, racial and sex groups. To what extent these vastly different patterns are a variable expression of the same condition or, conversely, represent completely different diseases remains unclear. The author favours the latter explanation, i.e. that several different disease entities are at present being classified as OA through ignorance. Similarly, pneumonia must have been difficult to understand before bacteriologists could identify pneumococci from mycobacteria.

The wide clinical spectrum of disorders given the same diagnostic label (OA) in rheumatological practice includes:

Epiphyseal dysplasias

Patients with epiphyseal growth disorders can present with premature 'osteoarthritis'. The correct diagnosis may be apparent from the family history and radiological changes, but the cause may not be clear in advanced disease confined to a small number of joints (Gibson and Highton, 1979). Minor degrees of dysplasia of the femoral head are thought by some to be a major cause of osteoarthritis of the hip (Solomon, 1976).

Ochronosis

Absence of the enzyme homogentisic acid oxidase leads to accumulation of homogentisic acid, and secondary polymerisation in the cartilage matrix. This can lead to premature joint destruction indistinguishable from idiopathic osteoarthritis. This rare genetic disorder therefore provides a model of osteoarthritis induced by a single biochemical anomaly. It has been suggested that a similar biochemical change may occur in ageing cartilage, with the accumulation of a pigment which might contribute to joint damage (Van der Korst *et al.*, 1977).

Chronic pyrophosphate arthropathy

A few people with chondrocalcinosis develop an aggressive form of osteoarthritis. This is characterised by a different distribution (knees, wrists, shoulders, hips) and special radiological features (patello–femoral new bone formation and large bone cysts), allowing it to be differentiated from other forms of the disease (Dieppe *et al.*, 1982). However, in many cases the correct diagnosis is not made. The significance of the mineralisation remains unclear, but it has been suggested that calcium-containing crystals may contribute to many other forms of osteoarthritis (Dieppe, 1982).

Generalised 'menopausal' nodal arthritis

All clinical rheumatologists are aware of this disease, which presents about the time of the menopause with inflammation in and around the interphalangeal joints (especially the distal articulation) and development of nodular swellings (Heberden's and Bouchard's nodes). As the condition advances, radiological

18

features of osteoarthritis become apparent, and other joint sites, especially the knees, may become involved (Kellgren and Moore, 1952). The aetiology and pathogenesis of this condition remains obscure, although genetic factors are known to be important (Stecher, 1955; Harper and Nuki, 1980).

Post-meniscectomy osteoarthritis

This is a well-characterised example of 'secondary' or post-traumatic osteoarthritis, and is fully described in the literature (Johnson et al., 1974). Of relevance to the present discussion are the very slow development of the disease, over decades rather than weeks, and the fact that only a proportion of patients are affected. This suggests that the changes may be multifactorial, and Doherty and colleagues (1983) have recently correlated the development of post-meniscectomy changes with osteoarthritis of the hand. Thus, secondary OA may depend on systemic predisposition as well as on traumatic stimulus.

Disease subsets at a single joint site

Epidemiological data show that osteoarthritis of the hip and hand behave differently, and are separate conditions (Wood, 1976). Recent information from a variety of sources suggests that several different patterns of disease can be recognised in hip OA alone (Brewerton et al., 1983; Marks et al., 1979). Similarly, a number of different clinical patterns are seen in osteoarthritic hands, although it is not clear whether these are due to different underlying diseases or to different manifestations of the same condition.

THE SYMPTOMS OF OSTEOARTHRITIS

As defined above, osteoarthritis is a condition affecting articular cartilage and subarticular bone. The cartilage has no nerve endings, and pain receptors are absent from subchondral bone (Wyke, 1981). It is therefore not surprising that OA can be asymptomatic. Lawrence's data (1963) suggest that only 50% of those with advanced OA (radiological grading 3 or 4) have articular symptoms, and that only 10% of those with early radiological changes will present clinically. Typical symptoms are outlined in Table I. The causes of pain in OA have been reviewed by Hart (1974) and by Harkness et al. (1983); they may include raised intra-osseous pressure, inflammation, joint instability, enthesiopathies, and the pain-amplification syndrome (Smythe, 1981). It is apparently necessary for some extra factor to develop, in addition to the changes in articular cartilage and bone, before symptoms appear.

This conclusion has relevance to the diagnosis and treatment of OA. The cause of symptoms must be explored as a separate issue from the radiological changes—and treated accordingly. Treatment of painful periarticular spots may have more immedi-

Table I. The symptoms of osteoarthritis

Pain: Various clinical patterns described (Hart, 1974)
Mild morning stiffness ⎫
Inactivity stiffness   ⎬   (Huskisson et al., 1979)
Immobility   ⎭
Symptoms are a late, variable feature of the disease, only present in a small proportion of those with radiographic change (Lawrence, 1963)

Possible causes of pain include:
Raised intra-osseous pressure (Arnoldi et al., 1980)
Tender periarticular spots (Dixon, 1965)
Inflammation (Dieppe, 1978)
Instability, with strain on the capsule, ligaments

From: Harkness et al., 1983.

ate relevance to the patient than therapy aimed at repairing the cartilage.

CONCLUSIONS

The human condition known as osteoarthritis is a common cause of pain and disability. However, it includes several different multifactorial diseases which share a late stage with similar pathological and radiological features. Symptoms are often absent in these diseases, and only develop if some additional factor is present.

Present knowledge of OA is scanty, being based largely on cross-sectional studies of relatively small numbers of patients. Many surveys concentrate on the hip joint alone, others probably include several diseases without being able to differentiate them.

The natural history of OA is not known, but it is likely that the clinical presentation is a very late feature. None of the changes develops quickly.

These problems make it particularly difficult and dangerous to apply data from animal models to the human situation. Changes in the cartilage are not analogous with the human clinical presentation seen by doctors.

Many of the problems presented by research on OA reflect the inadequacy of our clinical understanding. We do not know what questions the experimentalist should be asking. The direction of some of the present research efforts seems likely to need changing in the light of new clinical data.

REFERENCES

ALI, S.Y. (1978) New knowledge of osteoarthritis. *J. Clin. Pathol. (Suppl.)* **12**, 191–199.

ARNOLDI, C.C., DJURHUUS, J.-C., HEERFORDT, J. and KARLE, A. (1980) Intraosseous phlebography, intraosseous pressure measurements and 99M Tc-polyphosphate scintigraphy in patients with various painful conditions in the hip and knee. *Acta Orthop. Scand.* **51**, 19–28.

BREWERTON, D.A. (1983) Degenerative joint disease in the spines of patients with OA hips. *J. Rheumatol.* **10** (Suppl. 9), 34–35.

DIEPPE, P.A. (1978) Inflammation in osteoarthritis. *Rheumatol. Rehabil. (Suppl.)*, 59–63.

DIEPPE, P.A. (1982) Osteoarthritis and crystal deposition. In: *Scientific Basis of Rheumatology*, G.S. Panayi (Ed.), pp. 224–241. Churchill Livingstone, Edinburgh.

DIEPPE, P.A., ALEXANDER, G.J.M., JONES, H.E., DOHERTY, M., MANHIRE, A. and WATT, I. (1982) Pyrophosphate arthropathy: a clinical and radiological study of 105 cases. *Ann. Rheum. Dis.* **41**, 371–376.

DIXON, A.ST.J. (Ed.) (1965) *Progress in Clinical Rheumatology.* J.A. Churchill, London.

DOHERTY, M., WATT, I. and DIEPPE, P.A. (1983) Influence of primary generalised osteoarthritis on development of secondary osteoarthritis. *Lancet* **ii**, 8–11.

GIBSON, T. and HIGHTON, J. (1979) Muliple epiphyseal dysplasia: a family study. *Rheumatol. Rehabil.* **18**, 239–242.

HARKNESS, J., HIGGS, E.R. and DIEPPE, P.A. (1983) Osteoarthritis. In: *Textbook of Pain*, P. Wall (Ed.), pp. 215–224. Churchill Livingstone, Edinburgh and London.

HARPER, P. and NUKI, G. (1980) Genetic factors in osteoarthritis. In: *Aetiopathogenesis of Osteoarthritis*, G. Nuki (Ed.), pp. 184–202. Pitman Medical, Tunbridge Wells.

HART, F.D. (1974) Pain in osteoarthritis. *Practitioner* **212**, 244–250.

HUSKISSON, E.C., DIEPPE, P.A., TUCKER, A.K. and CANNELL, L.B. (1979) Another look at osteoarthritis. *Ann. Rheum. Dis.* **38**, 423–428.

JOHNSON, R.J., KETTLEKAMP, D.B., CLARKE, D.B. and LEVERTON, P. (1974) Factors affecting the late results after meniscectomy. *J. Bone Joint Surg.* **56**(1), 719–729.

KELLGREN, J.H. and MOORE, R. (1952) Generalised osteoarthritis and Heberden's nodes. *Br. Med. J.* **1**, 181–187.

LAWRENCE, J.S. (1963) The prevalence of arthritis. *Br. J. Clin. Pract.* **17**, 699–705.

MARKS, J.S., STEWART, I.M. and HARDINGE, K. (1979) Primary osteoarthritis of the hip and Heberden's nodes. *Ann. Rheum. Dis.* **38**, 107–111.

SMYTHE, H.A. (1981) Fibrositis as a disorder of pain modulation. *Clin. Rheum. Dis.* **5**, 823–832.

SOLOMON, L. (1976) Patterns of osteoarthritis of the hip. *J. Bone Joint Surg.* **58**(2), 176–183.

STECHER, R.M. (1955) Heberden's nodes. A clinical description of osteoarthritis of the finger joints. (Heberden Oration.) *Ann. Rheum. Dis.* **14**, 1–10.

VAN DER KORST, J.K., WILLEKENS, F.L.H., LANSINK, A.G.W. and HENRICKS, A.M.A. (1977) Age-associated glycopeptide pigment in human costal cartilage. *Am. J. Pathol.* **89**, 605–620.

WOOD, P.H.N. (1976) Osteoarthritis in the community. *Clin. Rheum. Dis.* **2**, 495–507.

WYKE, B. (1981) The neurology of joints: a review of general principles. *Clin. Rheum. Dis.* **7**, 233–239.

Chapter 2

Anatomical Changes and Pathogenesis of OA in man, with particular reference to the Hip and Knee Joints

D. L. GARDNER[1], R. MAZURYK[2], P. O'CONNOR[1] and C. R. ORFORD[1]

[1] Department of Histopathology, University Hospital of South Manchester, Manchester, UK, and [2] Department of Pathology, Medical Academy, ul. Unii Lubelskiej 1, Szczecin 6, Poland

SUMMARY

This review defines the zones of hyaline articular cartilage that are recognisable microscopically and describes the sequence of techniques by which synovial joints can be examined by pathologists. A definition of osteoarthrosis (OA) is provided and the abnormalities encountered in OA are distinguished from those encountered in ageing. An account is then given of the gross, microscopic and ultramicroscopic lesions of human OA, and a comment made on the companion processes of healing and of synovitis. Finally, a fully illustrated description is recorded of the abnormalities recognised at different stages in OA of the human hip and knee joints, comparing the acetabulum with the femoral head and the femoral condyles with the tibial plateau.

In the average adult human, there are nearly 200 freely moving synovial joints. They vary remarkably in their size, shape (Fig. 1), movement patterns and mechanical properties (Freeman, 1979; Gardner, 1986, 1987). Opposing bone ends are covered by avascular hyaline cartilage (Stockwell, 1979) devoid of lymphatics and nerve endings. The abundant cartilage matrix is synthesised by chondrocytes that are flat and ellipsoidal in the surface zone (I) but larger, ovoid and more often paired or in triplets in the mid and deep zones (II, III, IVA and IVB), as shown in Fig. 2 and Table I. Zone V is mineralised and firmly attached to the bony end-plate. Zones IVB and V are delineated and separated by a basophilic tideline which is often reduplicated, alters with time (Lane and Bullough, 1980) and marks a calcifica-

tion 'front' that is in a state of dynamic equilibrium. This structural heterogeneity is reflected in zonal variation in mechanical properties (O'Connor *et al.*, 1985b). The nutrition of articular cartilage comes from the highly vascular adjacent synovium and, increasingly in disease, from the subjacent bone. In both synovium and bone, nerves are frequent.

INVESTIGATION

Comprehensive pathological investigations of a human joint suspected of being the site of osteoarthrosis (OA) require that a sequence of radiography and photography accompany dissection. The radiographs and photographs provide a permanent record of the anatomy of the joint. Further photographs are likely to be necessary at each stage of the dissection, and all articulating surfaces are also recorded after the application of Indian ink (Meachim, 1972), which reveals fibrillary changes more clearly (Figs 3–14). Radiographs are conveniently made in a Faxitron cabinet, using fine-grain industrial or Polaroid film. Photographs can be made with any efficient macrophotographic equipment but, at additional cost, there is an advantage in using Polaroid apparatus with film that yields a negative. At suitable moments in the dissection, tissue is taken into liquid nitrogen

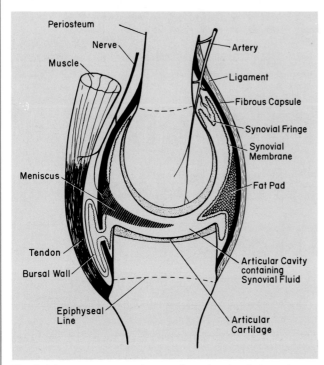

Fig. 1. Macroscopic structure of a synovial joint (based on the human knee).

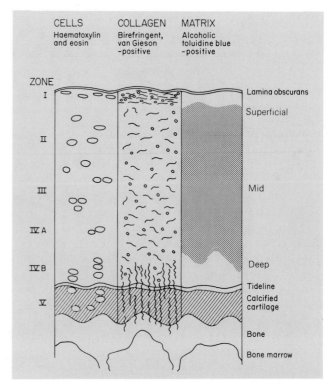

Fig. 2. Articular cartilage and underlying bone in a synovial joint, showing the microscopic structures revealed by different staining techniques: *Left*: Distribution and arrangement of cells in section stained with haematoxylin and eosin. *Centre*: Distribution of collagen fibre bundles in section stained with picro-Sirius red. *Right*: Concentrations of proteoglycans indicated by staining with alcoholic toluidine blue.

Table I. Zonal structure of articular cartilage (femoral condyle of dog)

Zone	Cells (haematoxylin/eosin)	Collagen content and orientation (picro-Sirius red)	Matrix: proteoglycan concentration (alcoholic toluidine blue)
Superficial*			
I	Single, ellipsoidal; small	+ + + + Tangential	+
Mid*			
II	Single, ovoid; larger than I; mean diameter 15–20 μ	+ + Random	+ +
III	Single, occasional pair; larger than II; mean diameter 20–30 μ	+ Random	+ + +
Deep*			
IV A	Single or paired; short columns; larger than III; mean diameter 30–40 μ	+ Random	+ + + +
IV B	As in IV A; short columns of 2–4 cells	+ + + Perpendicular	+ +

*Although convenient, this terminology is highly simplistic.

78°K (-196°C) or on to dry ice 208°K (-65°C) for chemical analysis, into nitrogen slush 63°K (-210°C) for low temperature electron microscopy, into neutral buffered formalin at ambient temperatures $c.$ 293°K (20°C) for light microscopy and into glutaraldehyde at 277°K (4°C) for conventional scanning (SEM) and transmission (TEM) electron microscopy. It is essential to standardise the techniques used for preparation of specimens, which are summarised in Diagram 1.

DEFINITION

Serious attempts are now being made to establish clinical definitions of OA (Gardner, 1983a and b; Gardner *et al.*, 1983b; Howell and Talbot, 1981) that will form acceptable criteria for the testing of anti-OA therapy (Altman *et al.*, 1983, 1986).

Osteoarthrosis is a collective term for the molecular, mechanical and functional deterioration and failure of the hyaline articular cartilage of synovial (diarthrodial) joints in excess of those changes that occur naturally with advancing age. The alternative designation 'osteoarthritis' is still widely used, particularly by those who believe that inflammation can play a significant primary role in the pathogenesis of OA. Osteoarthrosis does not affect the non-articular cartilages of the ear, nose and larynx; nor is it a disorder of non-cartilaginous fibrous and fibrocartilaginous joints in man. Nevertheless, these structures do undergo age changes. Osteoarthrosis is not confined to upright, bipedal hominids but affects other primates and many, if not all, other mammals, both surviving and extinct. The epidemiology of the human disease continues to pose intriguing problems (Acheson, 1983).

Hyaline cartilage is only one part of the bone-cartilage-synovial fluid-cartilage-bone continuum that constitutes a

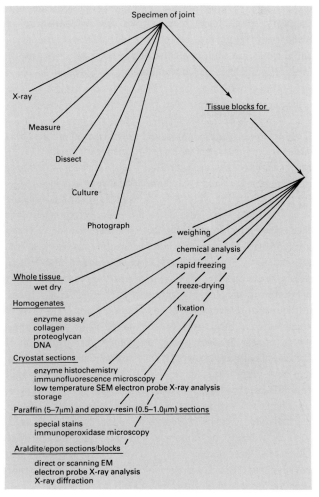

Diagram 1. Pathological investigation of a peripheral joint.

23

diarthrodial articulation. In any discussion of OA, synovial fluid, synovial tissue and bone must therefore all be taken into account together with the muscles that act across the joint, the tendons, the ligaments that facilitate the application of muscular forces, the capsular and periarticular tissues and the labra, menisci and discs that make normal joint function possible. Osteoarthrosis of the spinal apophyseal joints is distinguished from degenerative spinal joint disease, or spondylosis, a wider term that embraces changes in the non-synovial joints. Degeneration of the *fibrocartilaginous* intervertebral joints does not constitute OA, although systematic dissection shows that degenerative changes of the discs and apophyseal joint OA are almost constant associations.

In the final analysis, the disorganisation and loss of cartilage as a biological material in OA is attributable directly or indirectly to impairment or loss of chondrocyte function and/or to an inability by surviving chondrocytes to reconstitute the disabled tissue. At present, concepts of the nature and pathogenesis of OA remain very broad, and it continues to be helpful to think of OA as 'joint failure' in much the same way that we think of 'heart failure' or 'liver failure'. Advances in the genetics, biochemistry, physiology, biomechanics and ultrastructure of hyaline cartilage are now taking place with increasing frequency and it is not too soon to emphasise the sub-categories (pp. 18, 19 and 25) of OA to which attention must be directed.

AGE CHANGES

Osteoarthrosis is additional to, and superimposed on, the alterations in joints that occur with age (Freeman and Meachim, 1979). Much attention has been directed to age changes in articular cartilage (Gardner and O'Connor, 1986). With advancing age, the cartilage of the femoral head becomes thicker during the period of maturation from 20 to 50 years, before senescence accelerates. Mechanical compliance of the articular cartilage increases with age but creep compliance does not increase correspondingly. Tensile stiffness, fracture strength and fatigue resistance deteriorate. There is a rise in the content of water in midzone cartilage, presumably associated either with a change in the spatial relationships of the proteoglycans (PG), or with an alteration in their structure. The altered spatial relationships can, of course, be attributed to preliminary disorganisation of the crucial collagen–proteoglycan structure. Disorders of collagen have been held to contribute to defective tensile strength and resistance to shear, and defective PG to impaired compressive strength. A vicious circle is established; the ageing cartilage, mechanically prejudiced, responds to normal diurnal peak loads, such as walking, by abnormal and increasing deformation. Ultimately, these normal forces provoke mechanical failure and collagen fracture so that irreversible cartilage breakdown ensues with the onset of fibrillation (see opposite page).

The macroscopic age changes to which human synovial joints

are prone have been carefully recorded by Meachim and his colleagues, as outlined below. Those of the hip joint have been analysed by Byers et al. (1970). Much less is known of the intimate, microscopic alterations of hyaline articular cartilage with age than of the macroscopic changes (Byers et al., 1977; Gardner, 1986) but the small number of electron microscopic studies have yielded results of great interest.

The most obvious, gross change in human articular cartilage with age is the assumption of a yellow colour, with diminished translucency. Meachim recorded the surface topography and morphology of the patello–femoral joint (Emery and Meachim, 1973), of the ankle (Meachim, 1975), of the shoulder and hip joint cartilages (Meachim and Emery, 1973) and of the lateral tibial plateau (Meachim, 1976). The extent of intact cartilage, and of areas displaying minimal fibrillation, overt fibrillation, bone exposure and osteophytosis were mapped and measured. Other features such as 'parallel line' patterns of minimal fibrillation, 'ravines', smooth-surfaced destructive thinning, peripheral fibrous covering and localised incomplete defects were variously recorded for individual joints. For further details, the reader is referred to Meachim's papers.

The data accumulated by Meachim and by Byers et al. (1970) form a basis for anatomical accounts of articular change in human OA. Though by no means complete or comprehensive, they are indispensable guides to the investigation of the shoulder, hip, knee and ankle joints of ageing man and cannot be overlooked in any serious approach to the progressive lesions of OA which are not necessarily age-related but affect joints in which age changes are frequent. The age distribution of grade III and grade IV OA among over 1000 joints is shown in Table II.

Table II. Frequency (per cent) of grade III and grade IV osteoarthrosis by age in 1060 joints from patients over 50 (Collins, 1949)

Joints	Age (years) 50–59	60–69	70–79
Knee	2·6	12·0	33·3
Shoulder	2·6	9·7	15·7
Hip	2·7	12·2	16·7
Elbow	5·2	10·5	15·5
Great toe	7·9	13·7	18·2
Acromio-clavicular	1·3	9·6	12·3
Sterno-clavicular	1·1	1·5	7·0

THE UNIT LESION

In analysing any disease process, it is helpful to define a unit of pathological injury. The unit lesion of OA is an area of surface roughening of articular cartilage recognisable with the *naked eye* (Meachim and Stockwell, 1979). This lesion is termed descriptively *fibrillation*. Its recognition is considerably facilitated by painting the surface of the cartilage with an isotonic suspension of Indian ink, preferably free of phenol. The ink is applied gently but in abundance by a camel-hair paint brush. If the application is made to a moist surface which is then immediately rinsed with normal saline, very little carbon is retained even by overtly fibrillated surfaces. If, however, the surface is initially drier, and the applied carbon is wiped away with paper tissues, definition is improved and the minimal lesion is easily recognised. Photography is then readily undertaken. Recognition of the unit lesion of minimal fibrillation is also facilitated by use of a hand lens, a dissecting microscope or an operating microscope. The carbon applied to the articular surface is retained to a sufficient degree during fixation, dehydration, embedding and microtomy to be identifiable by TEM (Meachim, 1972); it is further recognised by conventional SEM but its presence does not preclude further study by SEM and histology (Brereton and Pidd, 1985).

CATEGORIES

Two classes of OA can be recognised, although the distinction may not be easy (Doherty *et al.*, 1983).

In the first, a substantial but diminishing group of individuals manifests material failure of hyaline cartilage without evidence of metabolic anomaly or endocrine disorder and with no history of infection or injury. In these persons, OA is said to be *primary* or idiopathic; its natural history is outlined in Diagram 2. One particular category, primary generalised OA (Kellgren *et al.*, 1963), occurs relatively often in older women and is heritable as a dominant characteristic. Primary generalised OA is much less common in men. The most frequently involved joints are the proximal and distal interphalangeals of the hands, the first carpometacarpal, the cervical and lumbar spine, the knees and the first metatarsophalangeal: other articulations are spared. It is convenient to use the term 'primary' to include not only the cases of primary generalised disease outlined above but also all other mono- or polyarticular cases where no cause is demonstrable.

In the second class, OA can be shown to have been caused by injury, infection, nutritional or metabolic disorder, endocrine dysfunction or other insult. Furthermore, the structure and function of cartilage may be prejudiced by congenital deformity of the whole joint or skeleton, and the underlying cause of deformity or metabolic disease may be heritable. Fractures involving articular surfaces, suppurative and tuberculous arthritis, rickets, gout, acromegaly and rheumatoid arthritis are among the numerous disorders that may be complicated by *secondary* OA.

At the present time, there is no clinical, chemical or morphological criterion by which the microscopic tissue changes of primary and secondary OA can be distinguished. Equally, there is no criterion, other than a reported difference in anatomical distribution, by which the early microscopic changes of primary

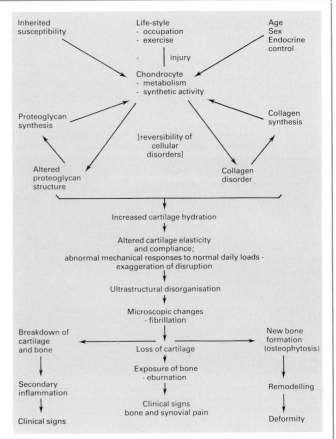

Diagram 2. The natural history of idiopathic osteoarthrosis.

or secondary OA can be distinguished from the exceedingly frequent, non-progressive cartilage changes of ageing. It is also noteworthy that virtually all forms of experimental OA are secondary (Adams and Billingham, 1982) although, under some circumstances, it could be argued that the articular changes of certain animal strains with spontaneous OA are primary. However, in the Labrador retriever dogs studied by Lust and Summers (1981), the OA follows the onset of hip dysplasia.

Table III. Pathological grades of osteoarthrosis in man

I	Patches of fibrillation or softening in central areas of articular cartilage, i.e. those not displaying simple age changes **Clinically silent**
II	Fibrillation more pronounced; early marginal chondro-osteophytosis with related synovial hyperplasia **Early symptoms**
III	Changes more severe; commencing exposure of subarticular bone and more generalised synovial disease. Osteophytosis **Usually symptomatic**
IV	Extensive cartilage loss and bone exposure; eburnation and bone grooving. Destruction of intra-articular ligaments. Fibrosis or atrophy of synovial fringes. Limb shortening, subluxation **Severe disability**

(After Collins, 1949).

GROSS ANATOMY

The overt lesions of OA (Table III) have been described in detail (Collins, 1949; Sokoloff, 1969; Jaffe, 1972; Ball *et al.*, 1978); the characteristic changes, showing the range of abnormality in the hip and knee joints, are illustrated in Figs 3–32 (taken during a one-year study of hospital necropsies). Osteoarthrosis culminates in full-thickness cartilage loss, bone exposure and eburna-

tion, remodelling and osteophytosis, cyst formation and the synovial uptake of fragments of cartilage and bone. Although isotope scanning techniques often reveal increased bloodflow at OA sites, this is probably an index of the increased metabolic activity of cartilage and bone cells in active disease and of the associated secondary synovitis, rather than a primary disorder. However, new bone formation by osteophytes is an early manifestation of experimental OA, and a substantially raised articular bloodflow could be one explanation.

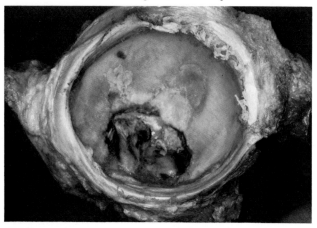

Fig. 3. Acetabulum. Note circumferential acetabular labrum and central zone of origin of ligamentum teres. Detail of surrounding, partly fibrillated cartilage difficult to ascertain.

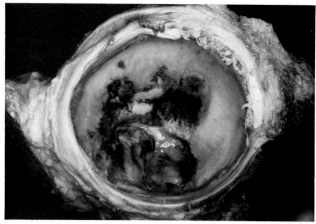

Fig. 4. Same specimen after painting with Indian ink: details of overtly fibrillated zones readily identifiable.

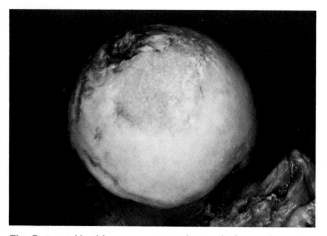

Fig. 5. Femoral head from same patient. Adjoining the fovea and occupying a considerable part of the upper, load-bearing area is an ill-defined zone of overt fibrillation, just distinguishable from the surrounding intact hyaline articular cartilage.

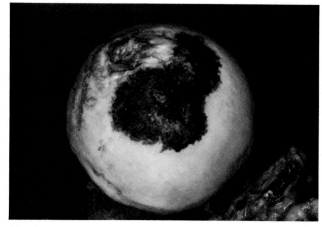

Fig. 6. Same specimen after painting with Indian ink: fibrillated zone of osteoarthrosis is readily seen and distinguished from softened area around fovea.

Figs 3–6. Hip joint, female aged 79 years. Paired photographs are provided to show the matched articulating surfaces of the acetabulum (*top*) and femoral head (*bottom*) of an elderly person. The value of painting with Indian ink is demonstrated: the ink is retained in fibrillated (roughened) zones of cartilage, enhancing the photographic contrast and enabling early detection, postmortem or at arthroplasty, of early or limited abnormalities.

HISTOLOGY

The microscopic changes characteristic of OA, illustrated in Figs 33–38, have been described very fully (Collins, 1949; Sokoloff, 1969; Ball *et al.*, 1978; Gardner, 1987). The covert lesions are: reduction in stainable PG; minimal fibrillation; collagen crimping; chondrocyte multiplication or migration, to form clones (chondrones); loss of cartilage; bone hyperplasia; bone exposure; osteophytosis; pseudocyst formation; and secondary synovitis.

The characteristic lesion, fibrillation, is not pathognomonic since it is a common structural result of molecular and ultrastructural disorders that can be brought about by many mechanisms, including the ageing process. In fibrillation, increasingly deep clefts form in the cartilage, and nearby matrix is depleted of metachromatic material. The path of the splits may be deter-

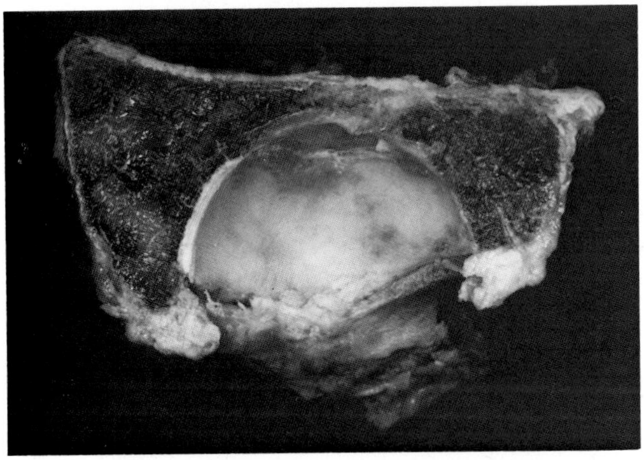

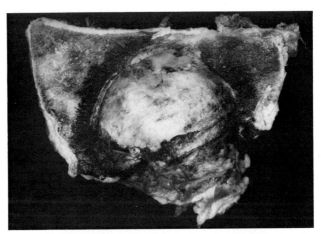

Fig. 7. Acetabulum, bisected to reveal apparently intact articular cartilage and subjacent bone.

Fig. 8. Same specimen, painted with Indian ink to reveal ill-defined, patchy, early fibrillation.

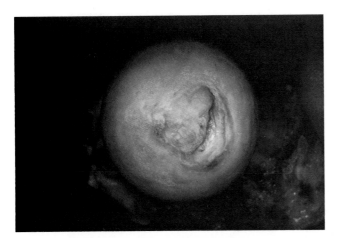

Fig. 9. Femoral head from same patient. With the exception of the perifoveal region, much of the femoral head appears intact.

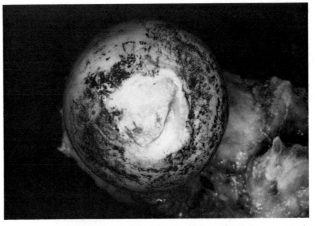

Fig. 10. Same specimen painted with Indian ink reveals that a surprisingly large proportion of the femoral head is the site of patchy, early fibrillation.

Figs 7–10. Hip joint, female aged 85 years. Compare with Figs 3–6. Paired photographs demonstrate the structure of the bisected acetabulum (*top*) and of the femoral head (*bottom*). *At left*, the articulating surfaces of the hip joint are displayed. *At right*, the same surfaces have been photographed after painting with Indian ink.

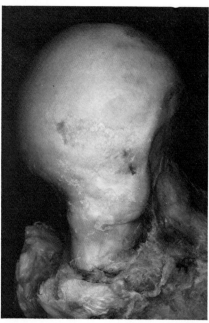

Fig. 11. Male of 66. Early, progressive fibrillation of osteoarthrosis extending over the inferior part of the head not normally affected by age-related change.

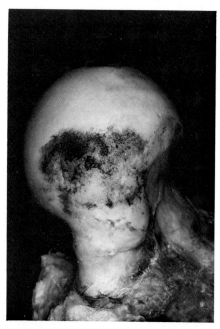

Fig. 12. Same specimen after painting with Indian ink: zone of fibrillation is readily distinguished from less severely affected cartilage.

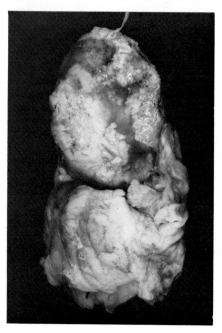

Fig. 13. Femoral head from female of 74. In the most advanced stages of osteoarthrosis, cartilage loss, bone remodelling and osteophytosis culminate in grotesque, mushroom-shaped deformity.

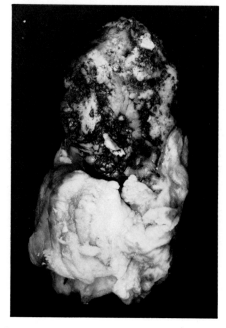

Fig. 14. Same specimen painted with Indian ink, showing that cartilage destruction is virtually complete.

Figs 11–14. Femoral heads: advanced osteoarthrosis in male and female. Such lesions are commonly encountered in specimens removed at arthroplasty. The value of painting fresh, unfixed articulating surfaces with Indian ink is demonstrated. Compare Fig. 11 with Fig. 12, and Fig. 13 with Fig. 14.

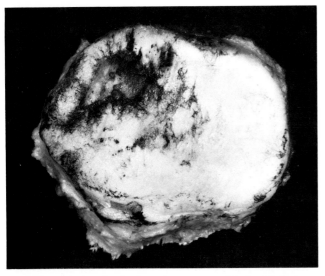

Fig. 15. Patella from female of 68. After painting with Indian ink, the larger, lateral surface shows severe fibrillation progressing to partial cartilage loss. The smaller medial surface is relatively spared.

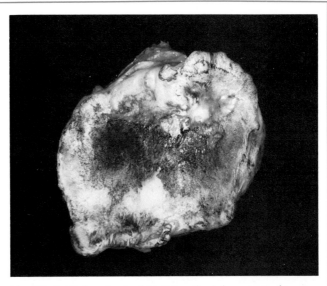

Fig. 16. Patella from female of 86. Osteoarthrosis has progressed to gross bone remodelling with large, marginal osteophytes. Central parts of cartilage of lateral (*left*) and medial (*right*) surfaces display severe fibrillation after Indian ink painting.

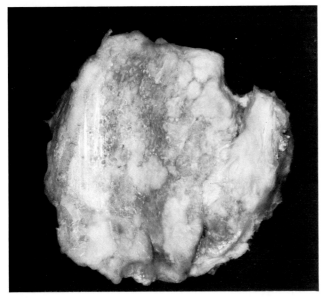

Fig. 17. Patella from female of 85. Loss of articular cartilage (*left*) has progressed to exposure of bone which has become eburnated and excoriated in lines of principal stresses. *Centre* and *right*: irregular cartilage loss, bone exposure and marginal osteophytosis.

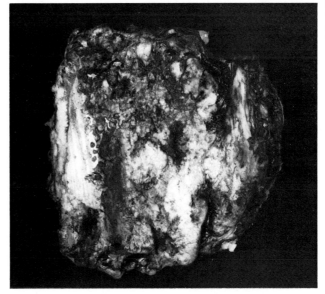

Fig. 18. Same specimen after Indian ink painting: the excoriated bone is seen as a relatively pale, striated white area (*left*) while the remaining parts show variegated pigmentation.

Figs 15–18. Knee joint: patellae, females aged 68, 86 and 85. Figs 15 and 16 demonstrate the severity of osteoarthrotic change that can be encountered in the patellar surfaces of elderly persons. Note the relatively slight disorganisation, in Fig. 15, of one bearing surface compared to the other. The disease affects different surfaces selectively for anatomical, mechanical and other reasons. Figs 17 and 18 emphasise the additional morphological detail that can be seen *naked eye* and recorded photographically after patellar surfaces have been painted with Indian ink.

29

mined by loci of weakness represented by chondrocyte lacunae rather than by the orientation of collagen fibres. Residual chondrocytes revert structurally and functionally to less differentiated forms and are often seen lying in groups assumed to be clones (termed brood-capsules or chondrones). Microscopic fibrillation is a late result of an earlier sequence of molecular disorders of the cartilage matrix; these, in turn, may stem from the initial alterations in chondrocyte function.

As the chemical structure of the matrix changes, a stage is reached at which the EM can detect morphological abnormalities. In time, these abnormalities become sufficiently severe to be visible with the light microscope.

Systematic light microscope surveys, of the human patello-femoral articulation for example, reveal a range of abnormalities from 'minimal fibrillation' to 'full-thickness cartilage loss'. The process is not uniform either topographically or in the time

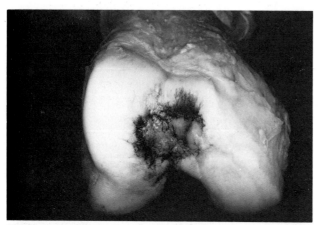

Fig. 19. Lower end of femur from female of 68. Overt fibrillation of central patellar surface has progressed to partial cartilage loss. Note apparent sparing of main condylar-bearing surfaces.

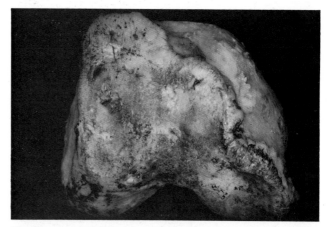

Fig. 20. Lower end of femur from female of 86. Widespread, progressive fibrillation and partial cartilage loss, seen after Indian ink painting, accompanied by formation of very large, prominent marginal osteophytes.

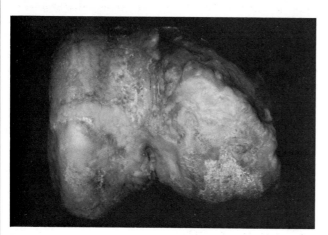

Fig. 21. Lower end of femur. The extent of fibrillation, cartilage loss and bone exposure is difficult to assess accurately in this unpainted specimen. Superficially, some of the patchy white deposits may readily be mistaken for the crystalline aggregates seen in chondrocalcinosis.

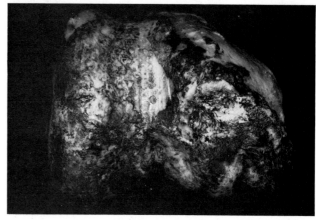

Fig. 22. Same specimen after Indian ink painting: exposed bone stands out as pale, grey–white areas streaked along lines of excoriation. Marginal osteophytes less readily seen but surface roughening and cartilage loss clearly depicted.

Figs 19–25. Knee joint: femoral condyles, females aged 68, 86 and 87. The bearing surfaces of the condyles shown in Fig. 19 are relatively spared: only the intercondylar, patellar groove shows overt osteoarthrosis. In the fresh specimen, however, the cartilages would have revealed the yellow colouration of advancing age. Figs 21 and 22 contrast the appearance obtained without and with Indian ink painting. Figs 23–25 are of the same specimen, rotated in the sagittal plane to show the distribution of osteoarthrotic change over all aspects of the femoral condyles and the extent of the osteophytes that have formed at the edges of bearing surfaces.

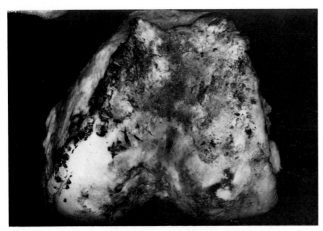

Fig. 23. Lower end of femur from female of 87. Indian ink painting reveals patchy nature of the widespread severe fibrillation with cartilage loss and marginal osteophyte formation. The changes particularly affect the patellar groove.

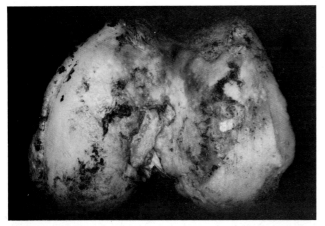

Fig. 24. Same specimen rotated posteriorly, to reveal the main condylar bearing surfaces. Bone exposure is accompanied by excoriation of the lateral condyle (*right*). Large osteophytes are seen (*left*) at the periphery of the medial condyle.

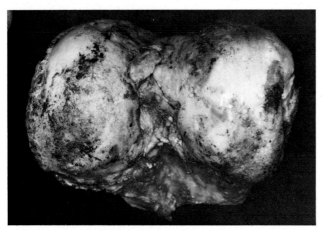

Fig. 25. Same specimen after further rotation, revealing the posterior aspects of the condylar bearing surfaces and showing the extremely variegated pattern obtained after Indian ink painting in grade III osteoarthrosis.

sequence of its development. Comparable surveys of the shoulder and hip joints suggest that regions of fibrillation may appear as early as the second decade of life. The ankle joint also displays central 'minimal fibrillation' that extends with age but is resistant to the vertical wear of clinically demonstrable OA, while the bare area of the tibial plateau shows 'overt fibrillation' to a degree related to age, and to a much greater extent than the meniscus-covered periphery.

In human joints with progressive OA, examined after surgery or post mortem, cartilage changes are very often accompanied by microscopic bone changes. New bone forms at the articular margin and is covered by fibrocartilage, the new rim constituting an osteophyte. The bony end-plate is frequently osteoporotic. Horizontal splits often occur at the line of demarcation between calcified and non-calcified cartilage and may be the result of an abrupt change in stiffness.

Age-related fibrillation alone seldom advances to cartilage loss. In OA, by contrast, cartilage loss progresses. The thickened bone is exposed and is seen to be white and ivory-like; it becomes grooved and excoriated, and loss of bone culminates in exposure of the bone marrow (Collins, 1949). Osteophyte formation continues and may be exuberant. The destructive process is most rapid and most severe when the sensory innervation to the joint is lost, as it is in syphilitic taboparesis or in syringomyelia. Accelerated OA changes are provoked by corticosteroids and have been linked with the clinical exhibition of indomethacin.

The unit lesion is characteristic of OA, just as the identification of a microscopic granuloma with central necrosis, epithelioid cells, Langhans giant multinucleated cells and surrounding lymphocytes is characteristic of tuberculosis. However, just as the histological features of a tubercle can be caused by *Mycobacterium tuberculosis*, *Mycobacterium bovis*, or several related organisms, or even by killed bacteria or bacterial extracts, so fibrillation can result from mechanical or physical injury, enzymatic or degradative change, or the incorporation of extraneous material such as amyloid into the cartilage matrix (Bartley *et al.*, 1985). Equally, there is no microscopic way to distinguish the fibrillation of developing OA from the identical change that is the hallmark of the ageing process.

ULTRASTRUCTURAL CHANGES

Much has been learnt of human OA by both TEM and SEM. Access to fresh material is not easy but, as autolysis leads to very slow disintegration of cartilage PG (Carney, 1982), it is reasonable to assume that the fine structure of the non-cellular matrix changes equally slowly. Chondrocytes retain metabolic activity, and presumably ultrastructural integrity, long after the death of the individual. The characteristic ultrastructural changes are illustrated in Figs 39–48.

Transmission EM of thin sections of articular cartilage shows

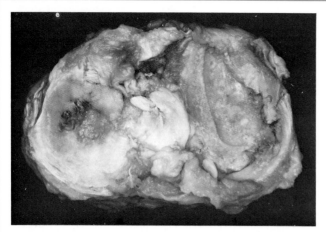

Fig. 26. Tibial plateau from female of 85. The atrophic and partly fragmented menisci are *in situ*. The inner rim of the lateral meniscus (*left*) is fissured and the central, hyaline-cartilage-bearing area roughened. The hyaline cartilage of the central bearing area of the medial condyle (*right*) displays incomplete, whole-thickness cartilage loss. The meniscus (incised during removal) is poorly preserved.

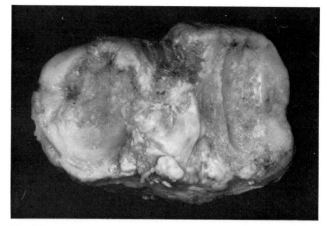

Fig. 27. Same specimen after removal of menisci to expose the submeniscal, hyaline cartilage. The peripheral hyaline cartilage of the lateral condyle is relatively smooth compared to the central part. However, hyaline cartilage has been lost from most of the central non-meniscal part of the medial condyle and eburnated bone is exposed.

the early loss of the normal arrangement of collagen fibrils, increased scale and variability in collagen fibril diameter, and increased quantities of interfibrillar matrix and water. Microscars develop from condensates of collagen fibrils, and matrix vesicles become more numerous than in normal cartilage. Amianthoid fibres are seen (Fig. 41). It has been suggested that the vesicles may encourage crystal aggregates of calcium hydroxyapatite and produce structural weakness. Chondrocytes are not lost initially; they retain metabolic activity and later, where chondrones form between clefts, appear to be capable of division and increased matrix synthesis. However, where the collagen microskeleton is destroyed, such structural recovery is not possible. Weiss (1978; 1979) considered that in established OA there are two morphologically distinct clones of chondrocyte, the first with an intensely staining pericellular halo, the second without. The significance of this distinction is not yet clear. With time, as fibrillation advances, structureless, electron-dense material accumulates in the residual superficial matrix. Chondrocytes degenerate further, cytoplasmic myelin figures appear, and chromatin condenses. Ultimately, only scattered cytoplasmic and nuclear fragments remain.

Advances in labelling techniques, using dyes such as ruthenium red or cupromeronic blue in a critical electrolyte concentration technique (Orford and Gardner, 1984), now allow OA changes in matrix PG, as well as collagen disorder, to be analysed. Brominated toluidine blue offers another similar approach (Mitchell *et al.*, 1980), and TEM of platinum/carbon replicas made at very low temperature is beginning to be used to study surface PG in OA (Gardner *et al.*, 1983a). Early ultrastructural disorder in experimental OA has been shown at a time when the surface is still intact (Orford *et al.*, 1983; Stockwell *et al.*, 1983).

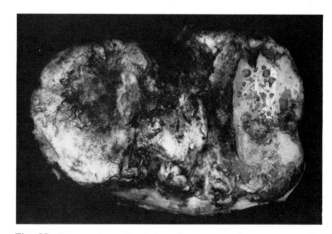

Fig. 28. Same specimen after Indian ink painting emphasises two main features: the relative integrity of the sub-meniscal, peripheral hyaline cartilage of the lateral condyle (*left*), and the extent of hyaline cartilage loss and bone exposure in the central part of the medial condyle (*right*).

The few published conventional SEM investigations of human OA confirm the presence and severity of the early lesions (Zimny and Redler, 1969; Redler and Zimny, 1970; Redler, 1974; Inoue, 1981). Many surveys have been made of animal material, notably in the dog (Ghadially *et al.*, 1977; O'Connor *et al.*, 1985) and mouse (Walton, 1977). New information has been gained by SEM of unfixed, hydrated material at very low temperature, a method that allows early alterations in matrix structure to be sought (Gardner *et al.*, 1981; O'Connor *et al.*, 1985a). In parallel with SEM studies, replication and Talysurf tracing have brought together measurements of increased surface irregularity in OA with loss of mechanical strength and elasticity, and increased deformability (Sayles *et al.*, 1979).

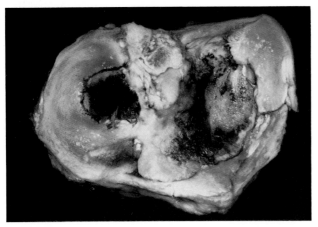

Fig. 29. Tibial plateau from female of 86, with menisci *in situ* and after painting with Indian ink. Note the deep pigmentation of the central bearing areas, the extent of fibrillation and the relative sparing of the meniscal surfaces.

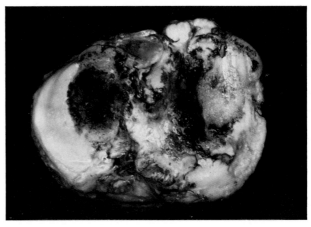

Fig. 30. Same specimen after removal of the menisci, showing very little roughening of the submeniscal hyaline cartilage of the lateral condyle; however, osteophytes distort the configuration of the medial condyle.

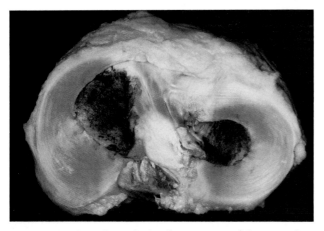

Fig. 31. Tibial plateau from male of 39, for comparison with Figs 26–30. Overt fibrillation of the central bearing surfaces of both condyles is shown by Indian ink painting. The menisci appear virtually intact in this younger male.

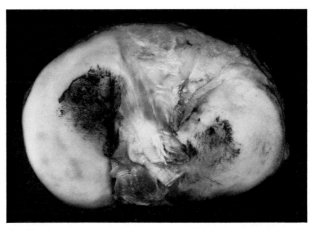

Fig. 32. Same specimen with menisci removed, showing the integrity of the submeniscal zones.

Figs 26–32. Knee joint, tibial condyles. Females aged 85 and 86 and male aged 39. In Figs 26–28, the relative distribution of osteoarthrotic change is indicated in relation to the menisci. In Fig. 26 the menisci are present; in Fig. 27 they have been removed. In Fig. 28, the contrasting appearances have been enhanced by painting with Indian ink. In Figs 29 and 30, a further example is given of the protection afforded by the menisci. The medial condyle is characteristically more severely affected than the lateral. These changes, of more modest degree and in a younger individual, are illustrated in Figs 31 and 32.

HEALING

Studies in healing (Vignon *et al.*, 1983) have revealed that repair in most tissues is by regeneration or by replacement fibrosis. Neither process is prominent in OA although, among the secondary reparative processes detected by Meachim and Osbourne (1970), fibrocartilage formation was relatively common. In the embryo, and in cell and organ culture of embryonic tissue, chondrocytes and their precursors avidly take up ^{3}H-thymidine, synthesise DNA, and divide. Chondrocytes in mature cartilage show no such mitotic activity but molecular substitution may be a mechanism of repair. In OA, human cartilage displays limited chondrone formation, often near the clefts of fibrillated zones. New formation of extracellular matrix is not adequate to balance loss, however, and the defects of OA appear to be permanent, although Bland (1983) questions this view. By contrast, there is collagen synthesis, PG change and an apparent increase in cell numbers in the dog model induced by surgical division of the anterior cruciate ligament. The explanation may lie in the severity of cell injury and loss in the human disease and the extent and irreversibility of the collagen destruction.

It is of interest to note that, when experimental cartilage defects are made, extending down to the subjacent vascular bone marrow, healing can take place by new formation of fibrocartilage. An analogy in man is the development of plugs of fibrocartilage that occasionally interrupt the surface of eburnated bone in grade III and grade IV OA; the plugs are in continuity with subchondral bone marrow. Experimentally, fibrocartilage formation is encouraged by continuous passive movement.

SYNOVITIS

Osteoarthrosis in man is regularly complicated by episodes of inflammation (Arnoldi *et al.*, 1980). Bone and cartilage fragments, liberated from degraded surfaces, undergo phagocytosis or lie within the synovia where inflammation is excited. The crystals of calcium pyrophosphate formed in the synovial fluid of older persons have a similar effect: their presence within cartilage prejudices its mechanical strength. However, low grade synovial inflammation in OA, without the presence of bone or cartilage fragments and without crystals (such as urate and pyrophosphate) visible by light microscopy, is commonplace among biopsies taken at late arthroplasty (Goldenberg and Cohen, 1978; Soren, 1978). The cause of this low-grade active inflammation continues to excite interest. One explanation, widely canvassed, for the synovitis of OA is the presence of calcium hydroxyapatite crystals that can be seen and characterised by SEM and X-ray microanalysis but are too small to be defined by light microscopy. Evidence that supports a further, more direct role for apatite crystals in OA has come from their demonstration in the cartilage matrix (Ali, 1980; Ali and Griffith, 1981). The inflammatory properties of crystals large or small, as a function

of size and shape, may also be exacerbated by the acquisition of a protein coat that can activate complement and lead to the production of inflammatory mediators such as prostaglandin E_1 and prostacyclin. Polymorphs, altered in this way, could be the source of elastase and other proteases able to break down nearby cartilage. Inflamed living synovia could also influence the integrity of adjacent cartilage via other systems, such as those in which catabolin (interleukin-1) is released, degrading the perichondrocytic cartilage matrix (Dingle, 1981). There can be little doubt that endogenous systems exist in synovia that can cause cartilage disintegration: whether these systems are *activated by* the progress of cartilage breakdown or whether, activated by other means, they *cause* cartilage degradation, remains uncertain.

THE HIP JOINT

This ball-and-socket joint, essential for normal human erect ambulation, is the most common source of the pain and disability resulting from OA. For these reasons the hip, particularly the femoral head, has been the object of numerous clinical, radiological, mechanical and pathological studies. Now that increasing proportions of ageing populations with symptomatic hip joint OA come to palliative surgery, femoral heads excised at arthroplasty are a ready source of material (Mankin, 1982). As a result, more is known of age and OA changes in the hip than in any other human joint.

The normal femoral head is largely covered by hyaline articular cartilage, which is not uniform in thickness (Armstrong and Gardner, 1977). The thickness of the femoral head cartilage increases with age linearly from 20 to 50 years; the thickest part, 20° anterior to the zenith in the latero-medial plane, increases to the greatest extent. There are also age-related changes in cartilage deformability (Armstrong *et al.*, 1979, 1980; Armstrong and Mow, 1982). As with the human femoral condyles, the articular cartilage of the femoral head is not normally smooth. Secondary irregularities, 0.5 mm in diameter and visible

Figs 33–38. Microscopic anatomy. Normal joint structure is three dimensional, complex and varied. The gross and microscopic manifestations of osteoarthrosis are even more diverse. Microscopically, the complexity is compounded at every level, from the light microscopic to the molecular. Figs 33–38 provide a few, two-dimensional impressions of the light-microscopic changes in osteoarthrosis of the hip and knee joints. The figures have been chosen to illustrate minimal (microscopic) and early disease in contrast to the late changes demonstrated in Figs 3–32. Haematoxylin and eosin (HE) shows the overall morphology. Martius-scarlet-blue (MSB) and picro-Sirius red (PSR) reveal the distribution of collagen (deep blue). Alcoholic toluidine blue (ATB) displays the distribution and changes in glycosaminoglycan and thus, by inference, in proteoglycan content.

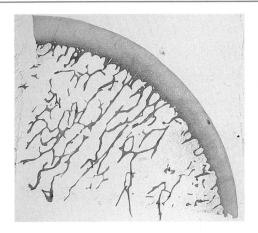

(a) Femoral head from female of 87. Normal hyaline articular cartilage, thicker towards zenith, with osteoporotic underlying bone. HE × 6.

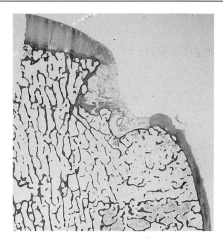

(b) Femoral head from female of 81, adjacent to fovea. Note irregularity (fibrillation) of thicker cartilage adjoining fovea. Underlying bone is osteoporotic and marginal cartilage much thinner than that near zenith. MSB × 6.

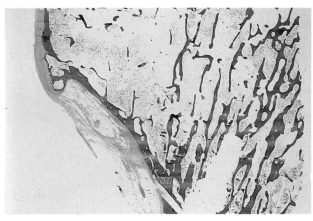

(c) Femoral head from female of 76, periphery. Small, early osteophyte with thin overlying hyaline articular cartilage. Osteoporotic bone structure. MSB × 6.

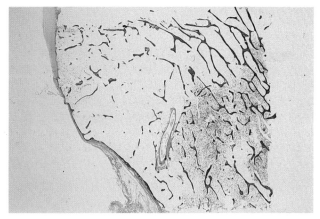

(d) Femoral head from female of 87. Field from periphery of same femoral head as (a), demonstrating well-preserved but thin hyaline articular cartilage overlying osteoporotic bone. MSB × 6.

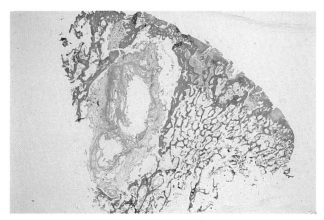

(e) Femoral head from an elderly person, showing gross mushroom deformity of osteoarthrotic femoral head with complete loss of hyaline articular cartilage, plugs of cartilage within superficial, exposed bone, and large central pseudocyst containing much loose, collagenous connective tissue. MSB × 6.

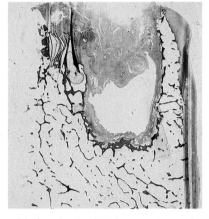

(f) Femoral condyle from female of 83 for comparison with (e). Note large pseudocyst within bone of load-bearing surface of lower end of femur. Part of the cyst is loose collagenous connective tissue containing blood vessels; part was fluid, shown as empty space. MSB × 6.

Fig. 33. Hip joint.

35

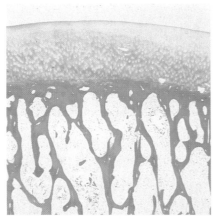

(a) Normal femoral head from male of 52. Note uniform structure of hyaline articular cartilage and well-formed, orderly underlying cancellous bone. HE × 14.

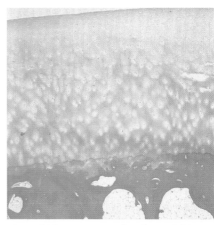

(b) Same section at higher power, revealing denser-staining, zone I cartilage and arrangement of chondrocytes. Note tide-line and relationship of calcifying cartilage to underlying bone end-plate. HE × 32.

(c) Same section at still higher power, for comparison with (a) and (b). Field embraces zones I, II and III and shows collagen-rich zone I, with the less collagen-rich zones II and III. Note distribution of eosinophilia in relation to chondrocyte lacunae. HE × 84.

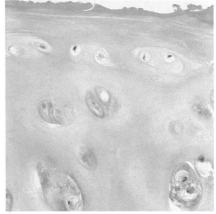

(d) Femoral head from female of 81, showing early fibrillation of hyaline articular cartilage. Note surface irregularity and inappropriately ovoid and round superficial chondrocytes. HE × 330.

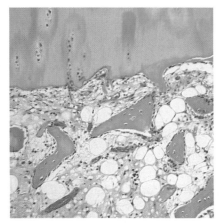

(e) Femoral head of female of 71. Osteoclastic bony reabsorption and appositional new bone formation in vascular zone deep into osteoarthrotic cartilage. Note numerous chondrones (*left*). HE × 130.

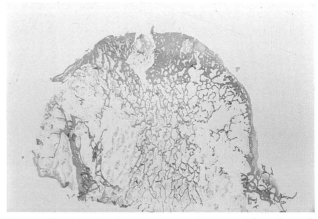

(f) Femoral head from female of 77. Extensive bone remodelling of severely osteoarthrotic femoral head. Note osteophytes at margin, central pseudocyst and loss of hyaline articular cartilage. Cyst lies at centre of zone of dense new bone. Remainder of cancellous bone is porotic. HE × 2.

Fig. 34. Hip joint

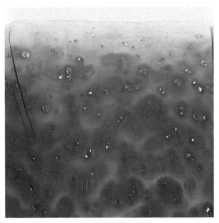

(a) Normal hyaline articular cartilage from femoral head of female aged 54, showing disposition of proteoglycan-poor zone I and proteoglycan-rich zones II and III. Alcoholic toluidine blue (ATB) × 84.

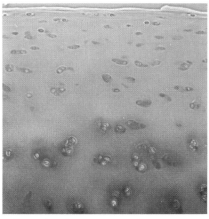

(b) Hyaline articular cartilage from femoral head of male aged 50, for comparison with (a). Artefactual lamina splendens (*top*). Polarised light. ATB × 160.

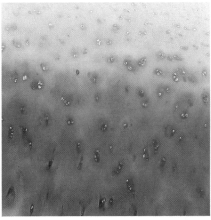

(c) Same patient as (b), for comparison with (a) and (b), showing early loss of proteoglycan from cartilage zone II. ATB × 84.

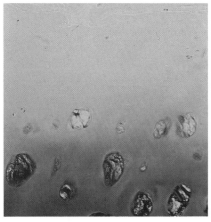

(d) Femoral head from female of 78. Fibrillation of disorganised cartilage surface overlying region of proteoglycan loss in zones I and II. Note well-preserved chondrocytes of zones II/III, where blue staining indicates proteoglycan retention. ATB × 330.

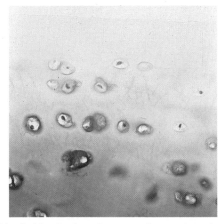

(e) Femoral head of female of 76, illustrating advancing loss of proteoglycan with retention of chondrocyte lacunae but variable staining for proteoglycans in and around cell territories. ATB × 330.

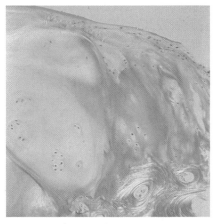

(f) Same patient as (d): marginal transitional zone demonstrating relationship of normal, peripheral collagen fibre bundles to edge of hyaline cartilage. Polarised light. HE × 130.

Fig. 35. Hyaline cartilage in osteoarthrosis.

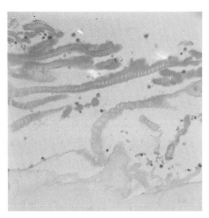

(a) Acetabulum from female of 78. Overt fibrillation, demonstrated microscopically by gross separation of collagen fibre bundles with loss of intervening proteoglycan. Polarised light. HE × 330.

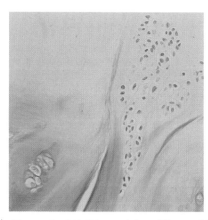

(b) Femoral head from male of 80. Between clefts and fissures of fibrillated cartilage lie islands (chondrones) of chondrocytes, multiplying in response to disorganisation. Note disparity in size between cells of chondrones and preserved chondrocytes of zones II/III of deeper cartilage. ATB × 330.

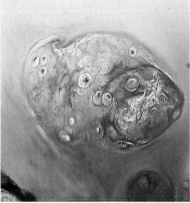

(c) Femoral head from female of 88. Island of divided chondrocytes, chondrones, in abnormal zone III cartilage at centre. No mitotic figures visible. ATB × 330.

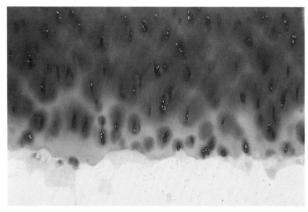

(d) Femoral head from male of 50, showing chondro-osseous junction. Upper part of field occupied by proteoglycan-rich cartilage of zone IVa. More deeply collagen-rich, less proteoglycan-abundant ridge of zone VIb tide-line delineates stained, upper part of field, in contrast to virtually unstained lower part where thin lamina of calcified cartilage adjoins bone. ATB × 84.

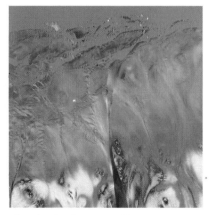

(e) Acetabulum from female of 78. Overt fibrillation with disorganisation of superficial collagen fibre bundles, some of which have assumed a crimped form. Polarised light. ATB × 84.

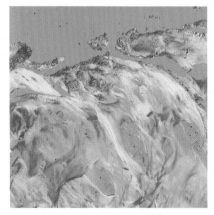

(f) Femoral head from male of 70, for comparison with (e), showing severe fibrillation that has not yet advanced to total cartilage loss. Changes shown in (e) and (f) would be readily recognisable to the naked eye. HE × 130.

Fig. 36. Cartilage changes in early osteoarthrosis.

38

with a hand lens, are superimposed upon the gross anatomical contours. An order of magnitude smaller are the numerous gently convex tertiary prominences, 20–40 μm in diameter, easily seen on the disarticulated surface examined by reflected light microscopy. Still smaller are the fibrous and non-fibrous irregularities that can only be detected when specialised forms of preparation, such as low temperature replicas, are examined by TEM (Gardner et al., 1983a). Vertical sections viewed by TEM show the presence of an amorphous, 500 nm, surface lamina (Orford and Gardner, 1985). These normal relationships are disrupted by the progressive abnormalities of OA, illustrated in Figs 3–14, 33–36 and 44–46; they must be distinguished from the limited fibrillation that develops with advancing age.

Systematic naked-eye studies of a large series of femoral heads obtained post mortem enabled Byers et al. (1970) to demonstrate that, as age advances, selected parts of the femoral head become roughened by fibrillation. The distribution of these fibrillated areas was also investigated in a Liverpool population by Meachim (1975); and Byers et al. (1970) and Meachim (1975) confirmed their location not only on the femoral head but also on particular parts of the acetabular surfaces. This pattern of age-related fibrillation, non-progressive in the sense that the extent and depth does not advance with age, can be regarded as a normal feature of the maturing adult human hip.

In addition to these common age-related alterations in hip-joint surfaces, Byers et al. (1970) found a distinct but uncommon pattern of deeper, anatomically progressive fibrillation with bone exposure and cartilage loss, affecting different parts of the femoral head and acetabular cartilages. These severe anatomically progressive changes were also identified in Meachim's studies: they were not clearly related to age and could be said to constitute the material failure of cartilage, and consequently to comprise the lesions of OA.

The advance of OA, with loss of articular cartilage, bone exposure and the marginal formation of new bone (osteophytes) covered by fibrocartilage, is accompanied by a gradual remodelling of the underlying bone structure. Horizontal clefts divide the calcified and non-calcified cartilage along the tide-line. Osteoclastic bone reabsorption and osteoblastic new bone formation culminate in grotesque malformation, and the femoral head may assume a mushroom-shaped deformity. Even before cartilage loss is complete in a vertical plane, the underlying bone has thickened by lamellar appositional new bone formation to such an extent that, on surface inspection, it may resemble ivory due to its pale colour and opacity. Bone, eburnated in this way, is an extremely inefficient substitute for hyaline cartilage as a load-bearing material: it is vascular, and nerve endings lie nearby. With movement, excoriation occurs and the coarsely scarred white bone surface breaks away, releasing fragments into the actively phagocytic synovium, provoking low-grade synovitis and exposing the vascular channels of the subjacent marrow.

Hip-joint OA is accelerated by the presence of concurrent infection, by continued occupational trauma, by the presence of crystals such as those of calcium pyrophosphate, by coexistent causes of inflammation such as rheumatoid arthritis, and by metabolic or endocrine dysfunction. Certain anti-inflammatory agents such as indomethacin have been suspected of exacerbating hip OA, perhaps by allowing tissue destruction to advance silently, leading to the need for early arthroplasty.

THE KNEE JOINT

This complex articulation is composed of two distinct bearing surfaces, the femoro-tibial, which has lateral and medial parts, and the patello-femoral. A pattern of normal, age-related fibrillation, common but not anatomically progressive, has been suggested by the detailed enquiries of Meachim (1976) and Emery and Meachim (1973); more severe, progressive lesions are also found. While loads borne by the femoral head are distributed over a significant part of the main bearing surface, loads on the convex femoral condyles are carried by areas that, in the normal erect adult, may be no more than 1.5 cm^2. Not surprisingly, the progressive changes synonymous with OA, and illustrated in Figs 15–32, 37–43 and 47–48, are often confined to particular parts of the joint.

Thus the patella is first affected (Collins, 1949). The patellar groove of the femur, the uncovered central parts of the tibial condyles, the anterior part of the medial femoral condyles, and the corresponding part of the lateral condyle are implicated in this order of frequency. The posterior parts of the femoral condyles, adjoining the median posterior recess, are little affected. Little weight is borne on the fully flexed knee and, in full flexion, the forces exerted upon the knee joint tend to separate the articular surfaces. Valgus and varus deformities of the knee are among the many local or regional diseases that predispose to OA.

PATHOGENESIS

Studies of pathogenesis (Gardner, 1983a and b) have made it increasingly clear that chondrocyte behaviour provides the key to the progressive cartilage and joint degeneration of secondary OA. Inherited cell defects can determine impaired collagen composition or cross-linking; the consequent chondrodystrophies, dysplasias or osteogenesis imperfecta then predispose to OA. Faults in the lysosomal breakdown of glycosaminoglycans lead to the so-called mucopolysaccharidoses: OA may result. Environmental influences also prevent chondrocyte metabolism and synthetic activity, and innumerable mechanical, physical, endocrine, metabolic, immunological and inflammatory disorders that disturb hyaline cartilage structure and function can lead in this way to OA.

39

It is therefore not illogical to argue that the chondrocyte is the key to idiopathic, so-called primary OA. The possible mechanisms have recently been reviewed (Gardner, 1983a and b).

The part played by *inherited susceptibility* is not clear. Among *exogenous agents*, mechanical factors are suspected. Excessive loads may, of course, act on normal articular tissues, and in this way occupations such as coal mining and ballet dancing and sports such as water skiing and hard-surface jogging promote secondary OA. The effects of the diminished loads that result from space travel have also begun to attract attention (Hernandez-Korwo *et al.*, 1984). In idiopathic OA normal forces, such as those of walking, act on prejudiced material. One hypo-

thesis that has been put forward argues that:

With advancing age, human articular cartilage becomes less cellular and contains more keratan sulphate. There are alterations in PG size and aggregability. One consequence is greater deformability in response to normal, diurnal loads. Evidently, stiffness is diminished, a change that may be related to the altered water content of aged articular cartilage.

If normal cyclic loading is continued, repeated deformation is likely to lead to collagen microfracture. As Freeman proposed, collagen fracture, in turn, destroys the microfibrillar skeleton that defines PG domains. Further loss of

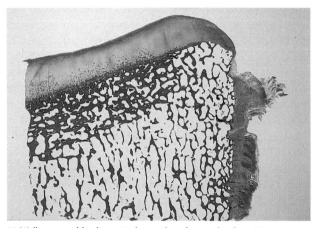

(a) Well-preserved hyaline articular cartilage from male of 50. Margin is zone normally covered by meniscus. Normally exposed, directly load-bearing zone lies towards centre (*left* of field). Note orderly surface, high collagen content of superficial cartilage zones, lower collagen content of deeper zones and well-formed bone structure. MSB × 6.

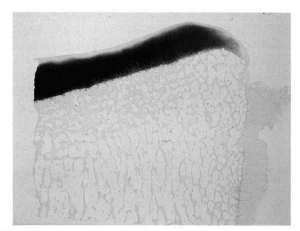

(b) Same tissue for comparison with (a), showing surface zone of well-preserved hyaline cartilage to be poor in proteoglycan, which is abundant in remaining zones II, III and IV. ATB × 6.

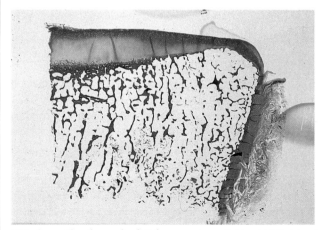

(c) Hyaline cartilage from male of 74, for comparison with (a) and (b). Peripheral hyaline cartilage (*right*), normally covered by meniscus, is smooth and orderly. Thicker exposed cartilage (*left*) displays early surface fibrillation. MSB × 6.

Fig. 37. Knee joint, medial tibial condyle.

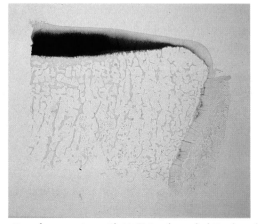

(d) Same tissue for comparison with (c). Proteoglycan depletion has advanced but is not confined to the fibrillated zone, suggesting that it may precede surface disruption. ATB × 6.

stiffness results in increasing injury. Cumulatively, ultrastructural damage may then begin, culminating in microscopic fibrillation and ultimately in progressive bone exposure. Broom and Marra (1985) suggest that loss of cross-linking between collagen fibrils is enough to cause cartilage softening.

Evidence to sustain this hypothesis, in which age changes in chondrocyte physiology are related to the progressive structural inadequacy of articular cartilage, may be obtained by programmed testing of aged, normal animal tissue.

There are other views. The role of bone in idiopathic human OA is suspect. Cartilage is very susceptible to repetitive impulse loading but is resistant to rubbing. The force of impacts sustained on walking downstairs, running or jumping is transmitted to adjacent bone structures which are strong, brittle and less deformable than cartilage. Normally, the thin cartilage lamina is spared the adverse effects of repeated impact by the energy-absorbing capacity of the bone but any change leading to increased stiffness of the subchondral bone may increase the susceptibility of articular cartilage to trauma caused by impact. It has been argued that bone may contribute to OA by undergoing stiffening as a result of numerous microfractures sustained before cartilage disorder is demonstrable.

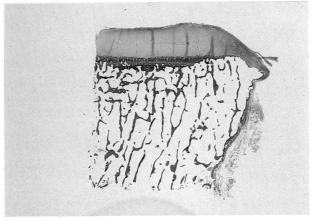

(e) Cartilage from female of 77 showing surface fibrillation across whole load-bearing area. Early changes indicative of marginal osteophyte formation. (Thickness of cartilage suggests that block may be eccentric; alternatively, fibrillation may have occurred marginally because of earlier meniscectomy.) MSB × 6.

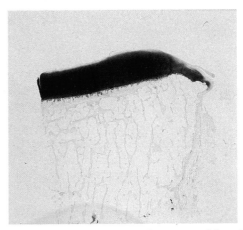

(f) Same tissue as (e). Deeply-stained proteoglycan preserved throughout zones II and IV, emphasising that observations in human material are not consistent or that more than one factor operates to promote fibrillation. ATB × 6.

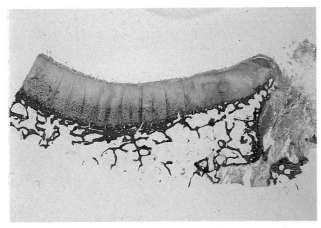

(g) Cartilage from male of 65, showing advancing fibrillation throughout the surface zone. MSB × 6.

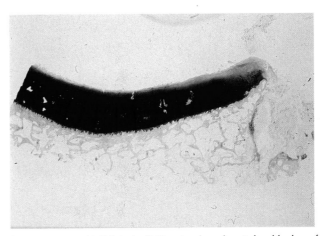

(h) Same tissue as (g). Relatively slight proteoglycan loss, indexed by loss of basophilia, with microscopic surface fibrillation. ATB × 6.

Fig. 37 (continued). Knee joint, medial tibial condyle.

41

CONCLUSIONS

Osteoarthrosis is a universal form of synovial joint failure common in humans and all mammals of both sexes, more frequent in older individuals but distinct from and superimposed on the changes due to senescence alone.

The unit lesion of OA is fibrillation which may be covert (microscopic) or overt (gross or macroscopic). The fibrillation that marks an early phase of OA is morphologically indistinguishable from the fibrillation of advancing age. Osteoarthrotic fibrillation is progressive: age-related fibrillation is not. In a commonly affected joint such as the hip, the presence of age-related fibrillation is usually identified in areas (such as the perifovear and marginal) distinct from those (such as the anterosuperior) where OA begins and advances.

Mammalian synovial joints thought to be affected by age or by OA should be carefully dissected with X-ray and photographic records at each stage to record the three-dimensional alterations. Sites selected in this way then provide material for microscopic, ultramicroscopic, analytical, and metabolic biochemical tests.

The heterogeneity of cartilage disease is emphasised. Since

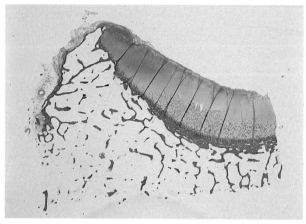

(a) Cartilage from male of 80, showing more severe fibrillation, particularly of central part of condyle (*right*). Note early new bone formation beneath central part of condyle. Ultimately, this sclerotic bone becomes exposed in the process of eburnation. MSB × 6.

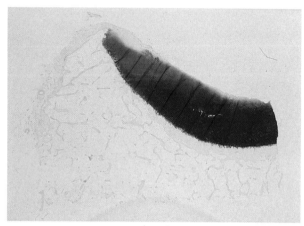

(b) Same tissue as (a). Note extent of proteoglycan depletion. The peripheral, transitional zone is always relatively proteoglycan-poor, and depletion here is greatest in this zone. ATB × 6.

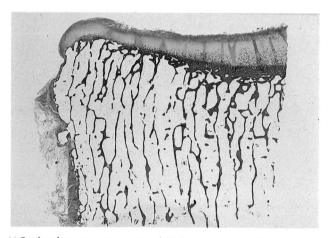

(c) Cartilage from same patient as (a) and (b), showing varying cartilage thickness and consistent fibrillation in *different*, compared with (a), but *adjoining* parts of condyle. MSB × 6.

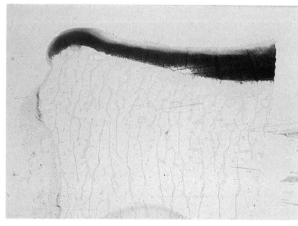

(d) Same tissue as (c). Note more extensive and more uniform proteoglycan loss than in adjoining part of condyle shown in (a) and (b). ATB × 6.

Fig. 38. Knee joint, medial tibial condyle.

a complex, non-congruent joint such as the knee requires to be analysed in three planes, against a time base, very complex considerations arise. These complexities mean that the comparison of joints from two normal individuals, genetically identical, in terms, say, of collagen type, content and disposition, is a very difficult exercise. When two genetically identical individuals are compared in terms of a single variable such as collagen at different times in the course of controlled, reproducible and standardised experimental disease, comparisons become even more uncertain. When attempts are made to extrapolate, in terms of, say, zones II and III of medial tibial condylar type II collagen,

from young, small, quadruped rodents, such as mice, to relatively older, larger, erect bipedal hominids such as man, then difficulties are introduced that require the most sophisticated forms of analysis.

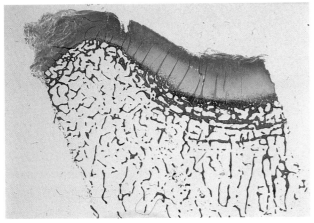

(e) Cartilage and underlying bone from male of 74. Advancing fibrillation leads to cleft formation. Deep ridge (*centre left*) probably artefactual. Underlying osteosclerosis despite evident osteoporosis of remaining bone. MSB × 6.

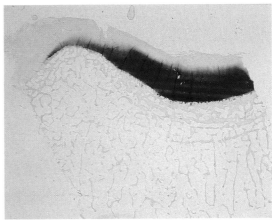

(f) Same tissue as (e). Widespread proteoglycan depletion, particularly severe at marginal, transitional zone. No particular relationship between degree of proteoglycan loss and extent of fibrillation. ATB × 6.

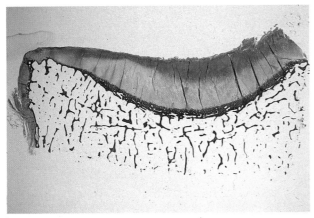

(g) Cartilage and underlying bone from female of 81. Note protection at lateral margin offered by meniscus (*left*), and advancing fibrillation (*right*) in part that is exposed and load-bearing *in vivo*. Underlying osteosclerosis of bone end-plate despite evident osteoporosis of remaining bone. MSB × 6.

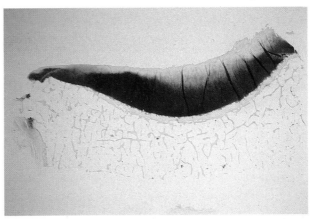

(h) Same tissue as (g). Widespread proteoglycan depletion, extending considerably more deeply than fibrillation. ATB × 6.

Fig. 38 (continued).   Knee joint, medial tibial condyle.

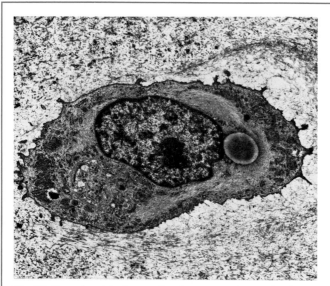

Fig. 39. Femoral condyle of mature dog, showing normal zone II chondrocyte, for comparison with Figs 40 and 41. Much of the cytoplasm is occupied by fine, intracytoplasmic filaments. Glutaraldehyde and osmium tetroxide; uranyl acetate and lead citrate × 5500.

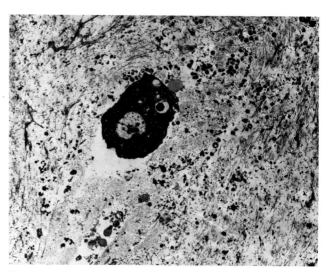

Fig. 40. Femoral condyle from (human) female of 64. Note remains of necrotic zone II chondrocyte from femoral hyaline articular cartilage. Glutaraldehyde and osmium tetroxide; uranyl acetate and lead citrate × 4100.

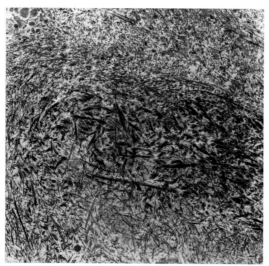

Fig. 41. Femoral condyle from female of 61. Accumulation of amianthoid fibrils, each up to 300 nm thick, in hyaline, condylar cartilage. Glutaraldehyde and osmium tetroxide; phosphotungstic acid, uranyl acetate and lead citrate × 5000.

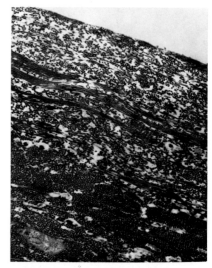

Fig. 42. Normal femoral condylar cartilage from female of 24. Note collagen fibrils closely packed, forming laminae arranged parallel to articular surface. Glutaraldehyde and osmium tetroxide; phosphotungstic acid, uranyl acetate and lead citrate × 7500.

Figs 39–48. Fine structure of osteoarthrotic cartilage shown by electron microscopy. The scales of magnification offered by the electron microscope (EM) are so much greater, on average, than those available to the light microscopist that it is difficult for the observer to cross the boundary from the first technique to the second. Nevertheless, many aspects of osteoarthrosis can only be approached and understood by EM techniques and it is therefore relevant to the present text to illustrate changes detected by transmission (Figs 39–43) and by conventional and low temperature scanning EM (Figs 45–46) and by low temperature replication in association with transmission EM (Figs 47–48). These latter techniques enable early microscopic changes of osteoarthrosis to be identified in unfixed tissue that still retains water.

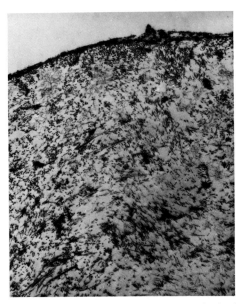

Fig. 43. Femoral condyle from female of 64. In this example of early 'molecular' osteoarthrosis, collagen fibrils are disordered in arrangement and widely separated, perhaps by matrix that is over-hydrated. Glutaraldehyde and osmium tetroxide; phosphotungstic acid, uranyl acetate and lead citrate × 8400.

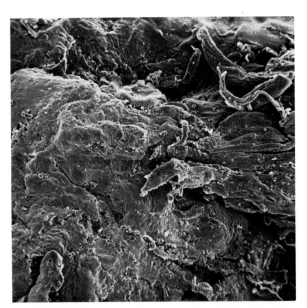

Fig. 44. Femoral head cartilage from female of 94. Fibrillation is established and would be readily recognisable by light microscopy at this stage. Note coarse separation of collagen fibre bundles. Glutaraldehyde-fixed, dehydrated, propylene oxide, vacuum-dried, gold/palladium coated and examined at ambient temperature × 147.

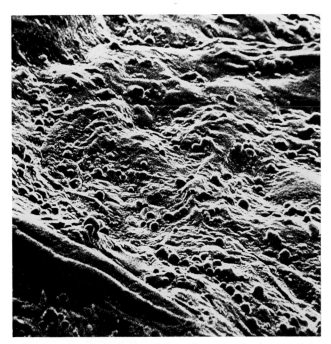

Fig. 45. Femoral head from female of 94. The degree of surface irregularity comprising fibrillation is shown in this hydrated specimen. Round and avoid prominences at surface may be chondrocytes or chondrocyte clusters. They are exposed during loss of proteoglycan and splitting (fibrillation) of associated collagen. Low temperature scanning electron microscope, nitrogen slush-frozen, gold coated and examined at 82 K (−191°C) × 200.

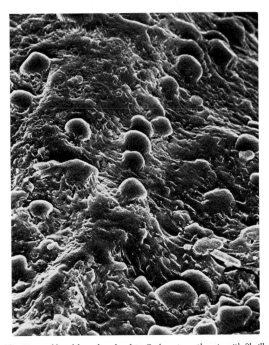

Fig. 46. Femoral head from female of 94. Early osteoarthrosis with fibrillation; surface of hyaline articular cartilage is punctuated by prominences (caused by chondrocytes) revealed at surface by loss of proteoglycan and disruption of collagen microskeleton. Note (*bottom right*) red blood cell confirming adequacy of hydration with minimal thermal damage. Nitrogen slush-frozen, gold coated and examined at 82 K (−191°C) × 638.

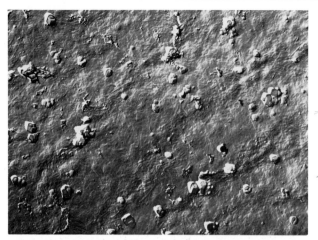

Fig. 47. Femoral condyle from normal *dog*. Hyaline articular cartilage surface demonstrating ridges 2–5 μm in width, on surface of frozen hydrated material. Freeze replication at 130 K (−143°C). Platinum-carbon replica × 4090.

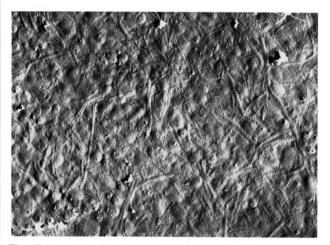

Fig. 48. Femoral condyle from normal *dog*. Compared with Fig. 47, articular cartilage surface displays banded collagen fibrils with a periodicity of approximately 70 nm. Between them lie 150–500 nm diameter rounded elevations, thought to be the surface representation of expanded proteoglycans. Freeze replication at 130 K (−143°C). Platinum-carbon replica × 9850.

ACKNOWLEDGEMENTS

The continued support of the Medical Research Council, the Arthritis and Rheumatism Council for Research, and Ciba-Geigy Pharmaceuticals is gratefully acknowledged.

REFERENCES

ACHESON, R.M. (1983) Osteoarthrosis—the mystery crippler. *J. Rheumatol.* **10**, 174–176.

ADAMS, M.E. and BILLINGHAM, M.E.J. (1982) Animal models of degenerative joint disease. In: *Current Topics in Pathology*, Vol. 71, C.L. Berry (Ed.), pp. 265–297. Springer, Berlin/Heidelberg.

ALI, S.Y. (1980) Mineral-containing matrix vesicles in human osteoarthrotic cartilage. In: *The Aetiopathogenesis of Osteoarthrosis*, G. Nuki (Ed.), pp. 105–116. Pitman Medical, Tunbridge Wells.

ALI, S.Y. and GRIFFITH, S. (1981) New types of calcium phosphate crystals in arthritic cartilage. *Semin. Arthritis Rheum.* **11** (Suppl. 1), 124–126.

ALTMAN, R.D., MEENAN, R.F., HOCHBERG, M.C., BOLE, C.G., BRANDT, K., COOK, T.D.V., GREENWALD, R.A., HOWELL, D.S., KAPLAN, D., KOOPMAN, W.J., MANKIN, H., MIKKELSEN, W.M., MOSKOWITZ, R. and SOKOLOFF, L. (1983) An approach to developing criteria for the clinical diagnosis and classification of osteoarthritis: a status report of the American Rheumatism Association diagnostic subcommittee on osteoarthritis. *J. Rheumatol.* **10**, 180–183.

ALTMAN, R.D., ASCH, E., BLOCH, D., BOLE, C.G., BORENSTEIN, B.D., BRANDT, K., CHRISTY, W., COOK, T.D.V., GREENWALD, R., HOCHBERG, N., HOWELL, D.S., KAPLAN, D., KOOPMAN, W.J., LONGLEY, S., MANKIN, H., McSHANE, D.J., MEDSGER, T., MEENAN., R.F., MIKKELSEN, W.M., MOSKOWITZ, R., MURPHY, W., ROTHSCHILD, B., SEGAL, M., SOKOLOFF, L. AND WOLFE, F. (1986) Development of criteria for the classification and reporting of osteoarthrosis—classification of osteoarthritis of the knee. *Arthritis Rheum.* **29**, 1039–1049.

ARMSTRONG, C.G., BAHRANI, A.S. and GARDNER, D.L. (1979) *In vitro* measurement of articular cartilage deformations in the intact human hip joint under load. *J. Bone Joint Surg.* **61**A, 744–755.

ARMSTRONG, C.G., BAHRANI, A.S. and GARDNER, D.L. (1980) Changes in the deformational behaviour of human hip cartilage with age. *J. Biomech. Eng.* **102**, 214–220.

ARMSTRONG, C.G. and GARDNER, D.L. (1977) Thickness and distribution of human femoral head articular cartilage. *Ann. Rheum. Dis.* **36**, 407–412.

ARMSTRONG, C.G. and MOW, V.C. (1982) Variations in the intrinsic mechanical properties of human articular cartilage with age, degeneration and water content. *J. Bone Joint Surg.* **64**A, 88–94.

ARNOLDI, C.C., REIMANN, I. and BRETLAN, P. (1980) The synovial membrane in human coxarthrosis: light and electron microscopic studies. *Clin. Orthop. Rel. Res.* **148**, 213–220.

BALL, J., SHARP, J. and SHAW, N.E. (1978) Osteoarthrosis. In: *Copeman's Textbook of the Rheumatic Diseases*, 5th edn, J.T. Scott (Ed.), pp. 595–644. Churchill Livingstone, Edinburgh.

BARTLEY, C.J., ORFORD, C.R. and GARDNER, D.L. (1985) Amyloid in ageing articular cartilage. *J. Pathol.* **145**, 107A.

BLAND, J.H. (1983) The reversibility of osteoarthritis: a review. *Am. J. Med.* **74**, 16–26.

BRERETON, J.D. and PIDD, J.G. (1985) The effect of India ink painting on the ultrastructural appearance of human hyaline articular cartilage. *J. Electron Microsc. Tech.* **2**, 515–516.

BROOM, N.D. and MARRA, D.L. (1985) New structural concepts of articular cartilage demonstrated with a physical model. *Connect. Tissue Res.* **14**, 1–8.

BYERS, P.D., CONTEPOMI, C.A. and FARKAS, T.A. (1970) A post mortem study of the hip joint including the prevalence of the features of the right side. *Ann. Rheum. Dis.* **29**, 15–31.

BYERS, P.D., MAROUDAS, A., OZTOP, F., STOCKWELL, R.A. and VENN, M.F. (1977) Histological and biochemical studies on cartilage from osteoarthrotic femoral heads with special reference to surface characteristics. *Connect. Tissue Res.* **5**, 41–49.

CARNEY, S.L. (1982) A study of the macromolecular biochemistry of articular connective tissue. PhD Thesis, University of Manchester.

COLLINS, D.H. (1949) *The Pathology of Articular and Spinal Diseases*, pp. 74–115. Edward Arnold, London.

DINGLE, J.T. (1981) Catabolin—a cartilage catabolic factor from synovium. *Clin. Orthop. Rel. Res.* **156**, 219–231.

DOHERTY, M., WATT, I. and DIEPPE, P. (1983) Influence of primary generalised osteoarthritis on development of secondary osteoarthritis. *Lancet* **ii**, 8–11.

EMERY, I.H. and MEACHIM, G. (1973) Surface morphology and topography of patello-femoral cartilage fibrillation in Liverpool necropsies. *J. Anat.* **116**, 103–120.

FREEMAN, M.A.R. (1979) *Adult Articular Cartilage*, 2nd edn. Pitman Medical, Tunbridge Wells.

FREEMAN, M.A.R. and MEACHIM, G. (1979) Ageing and degeneration. In: *Adult Articular Cartilage*, 2nd edn, M.A.R. Freeman (Ed.), pp. 487–543. Pitman Medical, Tunbridge Wells.

GARDNER, D.L. (1983a) The nature and causes of osteoarthrosis. *Br. Med. J.* **286**, 418–424.

GARDNER, D.L. (1983b) Is osteoarthritis a disease of ageing midzone chondrocytes? *J. Rheumatol.* **10** (Suppl. 9), 110–111.

GARDNER, D.L. (1986) Structure and function of connective tissue and joints. In: *Copeman's Textbook of the Rheumatic Diseases*, 6th edn, J.T. Scott (Ed.), pp. 199–250. Churchill Livingstone, Edinburgh.

GARDNER, D.L. (1987) *Pathological Basis of the Connective Tissue Diseases*. Edward Arnold, London (in preparation).

GARDNER, D.L. and O'CONNOR, P. (1985) The musculoskeletal system—ageing of articular cartilage. In: *Textbook of Geriatric Medicine and Gerontology*, 3rd edn, J.C. Brocklehurst (Ed.), pp. 776–794. Churchill Livingstone, Edinburgh.

GARDNER, D.L., O'CONNOR, P., MIDDLETON, J.F.S., OATES, K. and ORFORD, C.R. (1983a) An investigation by transmission electron microscopy of freeze replicas of dog articular cartilage surfaces: the fibre-rich surface structure. *J. Anat.* **137**, 573–582.

GARDNER, D.L., O'CONNOR, P. and OATES, K. (1981) Low temperature scanning electron microscopy of dog and guinea-pig hyaline articular cartilage. *J. Anat.* **132**, 267–282.

GARDNER, D.L., OATES, K., O'CONNOR, P. and ORFORD, C.R. (1983b) The microscopic heterogeneity of osteoarthrosis. *J. Rheumatol.* **10** (Suppl. 9), 9–10.

GHADIALLY, F.N., GHADIALLY, J.A., ORYSHAK, A.F. and YONG, N.K. (1977) The surface of dog articular cartilage. A scanning electron microscope study. *J. Anat.* **123**, 527–536.

GOLDENBERG, D.L. and COHEN, A.S. (1978) Synovial membrane histopathology in the differential diagnosis of rheumatoid arthritis, gout, pseudogout, systemic lupus erythematosus, infectious arthritis and degenerative joint disease. *Medicine* **57**, 239–252.

HERNANDEZ-KORWO, R., KOZLOVSKAYA, I.B., KREIDICH, Y.V., MARTINEZ-FERNANDEZ, S., RAKHMANOV, A.S., FERNANDEZ-PONE, E. and MINENKO, A.V. (1984) Effect of the 7-day space flight on the structure and function of man's bones and joints. *Kosm. Biol. Aviakosm. Med.* **17**, 37–43.

HOWELL, D. and TALBOT, J.H. (1981) Osteoarthritis Symposium. *Semin. Arthritis. Rheum.* **XI** (Suppl. 1), 1–149.

INOUE, H. (1981) Alterations in the collagen framework of osteoarthritic cartilage and subchondral bone. *Intern. Orthop.* **5**, 47–52.

JAFFE, H.L. (1972) Degenerative joint disease. In: *Metabolic, Degenerative, and Inflammatory Diseases of Bones and Joints*, pp. 735–778. Lea and Febiger, Philadelphia.

KELLGREN, J.H., LAWRENCE, J.S. and BIER, F. (1963) Genetic factors in generalised osteoarthrosis. *Ann. Rheum. Dis.* **22**, 237–255.

LANE, L.B. and BULLOUGH, P.G. (1980) Age-related changes in the thickness of the calcified zone and the number of tidemarks in adult articular cartilage. *J. Bone Joint. Surg.* **62**B, 372–375.

LUST, G. and SUMMERS, D.A. (1981) Early asymptomatic stage of degenerative joint disease in canine hip joints. *Am. J. Vet. Res.* **42**, 1849–1855.

MANKIN, H.J. (1982) The response of articular cartilage to mechanical injury. *J. Bone Joint Surg.* **64**A, 460–466.

MEACHIM, G. (1972) Light microscopy of Indian ink preparations of fibrillated cartilage. *Ann. Rheum. Dis.* **31**, 457–464.

MEACHIM, G. (1975) Cartilage fibrillation at the ankle joint in Liverpool necropsies. *J. Anat.* **119**, 601–610.

MEACHIM, G. (1976) Cartilage fibrillation on the lateral tibial plateau in Liverpool necropsies. *J. Anat.* **121**, 97–106.

MEACHIM, G. and EMERY, I.H. (1973) Cartilage fibrillation in shoulder and hip joints in Liverpool necropsies. *J. Anat.* **116**, 161–179.

MEACHIM, G. and OSBORNE, G.V. (1970) Repair at the femoral articular surface in osteoarthritis of the hip. *J. Pathol.* **102**, 1–8.

MEACHIM, G. and STOCKWELL, R.A. (1979) The matrix. In: *Adult Articular Cartilage*, 2nd edn, M.A.R. Freeman (Ed.), pp. 1–67. Pitman Medical, Tunbridge Wells.

MITCHELL, N., SHEPARD, N. and HARROD, J. (1980) The use of brominated toluidine blue 0 in X-ray microanalysis for proteoglycan. A new technique. *Histochemistry* **68**, 245–251.

O'CONNOR, P., OATES, K., GARDNER, D.L., MIDDLETON, J.F.S., ORFORD, C.R. and BRERETON, J.D. (1985a) Low temperature and conventional scanning electron microscopic observations of dog femoral condylar cartilage surface after anterior cruciate ligament division. *Ann. Rheum. Dis.* **44**, 321–327.

O'CONNOR, P., ORFORD, C.R. and GARDNER, D.L. (1985b) Role of proteoglycan and collagen in the mechanical behaviour of articular cartilage. *Br. J. Rheumatol.* **24**, 200.

ORFORD, C.R. and GARDNER, D.L. (1984) Proteoglycan association with collagen d band in hyaline articular cartilage. *Connect. Tissue Res.* **12**, 345–348.

ORFORD, C.R. and GARDNER, D.L. (1985) Ultrastructural histochemistry of the surface lamina of normal articular cartilage. *Histochem. J.* **17**, 223–233.

ORFORD, C.R., GARDNER, D.L. and O'CONNOR, P. (1983) Ultrastructural changes in dog femoral condylar cartilage following anterior cruciate ligament section. *J. Anat.* **137**, 653–663.

ORFORD, C.R., GARDNER, D.L., O'CONNOR, P., BATES, G., SWALLOW, J.J. and BRITO-BABAPULLE (1986) Ultrastructural alterations in glycosaminoglycans of dog femoral condylar cartilage after surgical division of an anterior cruciate ligament: a study with cupro-meronic blue in a critical electrolyte concentration technique. *J. Anat.* **148**, 233–244.

REDLER, I. (1974) A scanning electron microscopic study of human normal and osteoarthritic articular cartilage. *Clin. Orthop. Rel. Res.* **103**, 262–268.

REDLER, I. and ZIMNY, M.L. (1970) Scanning electron microscopy of normal and abnormal articular cartilage and synovium. *J. Bone Joint Surg.* **52**A, 1395–1404.

SAYLES, R.S., THOMAS, T.R., ANDERSON, J., HASLOCK, I. and UNSWORTH, A. (1979) Measurement of the surface microgeometry of articular cartilage. *J. Biomech.* **12**, 257–267.

SOKOLOFF, L. (1969) *The Biology of Degenerative Joint Disease.* University of Chicago Press, Chicago and London.

SOREN, A. (1978) *Histodiagnosis and Clinical Correlation of Rheumatoid and Other Synovitis*, pp. 116–122. J.B. Lippincott, Philadelphia and Toronto.

STOCKWELL, R.A. (1979) *Biology of Cartilage Cells*, pp. 245–247. Cambridge University Press, Cambridge.

STOCKWELL, R.A., BILLINGHAM, M.E.J. and MUIR, H. (1983) Ultrastructural changes in articular cartilage after experimental section of the anterior cruciate ligament of the dog knee. *J. Anat.* **136**, 425–439.

VIGNON, E., ARLOT, M., HARTMANN, D., MOYEN, B. and VILLE, G. (1983) Hypertrophic repair of articular cartilage in experimental osteoarthrosis. *Ann. Rheum. Dis.* **42**, 82–88.

WALTON, M. (1977) Studies of degenerative joint disease in the mouse knee. III. Scanning electron microscopy. *J. Pathol.* **123**, 211–217.

WEISS, C. (1978) Light and electron microscopic studies of osteoarthritic articular cartilage. In: *The Human Joint in Health and Disease*, W.H. Simon (Ed.), pp. 112–121. University of Pennsylvania Press, Philadelphia.

WEISS, C. (1979) Normal and osteoarthritic articular cartilage. *Orthop. Clin. North Am.* **10**, 175–189.

ZIMNY, M.L. and REDLER, I. (1969) An ultrastructural study of patellar chondromalacia in humans. *J. Bone Joint Surg.* **51**A, 1179–1190.

Chapter 3

Biochemical Changes in Human Osteoarthrotic Cartilage

M. T. BAYLISS*

Experimental Pathology Unit, Institute of Orthopaedics, Royal National Orthopaedic Hospital, Stanmore, Middlesex, UK

*Now at The Mathilda and Terence Kennedy Institute of Rheumatology, London.

SUMMARY

Among the changes in cartilage structure that characterise osteoarthrosis, the most consistent is a loss of proteoglycan, which is directly proportional to the severity of the lesion. Although the collagen content remains unchanged and there is no significant alteration in the types of collagen synthesised, there are qualitative defects in the collagen framework. These appear to be related to the swelling and increased water content of some osteoarthritic specimens. The significance of changes in proteoglycan metabolism are more controversial. Some studies have reported an increased synthesis, suggesting an attempt at repair, while others have shown normal synthesis rates. The ultimate loss of proteoglycan appears to be determined by catabolic activity in osteoarthrotic cartilage, in which there is considerable evidence of proteolytic enzyme activity capable of degrading proteoglycan and cartilage. Recent studies of all these changes are reviewed below.

Many studies over the last 40–50 years have attempted to define the morphology and histology of osteoarthritic articular cartilage. Collins (1949) described a scheme in which the earliest changes included: (i) loss of the surface layers of cartilage, (ii) a decrease in metachromatic staining, indicating a loss of proteoglycan, and (iii) penetration of the tide-mark by blood vessels. Since then there have been numerous investigations primarily concerned with biochemical changes in the macromolecules (collagen and proteoglycan) that comprise the extracellular matrix.

COLLAGEN

Although it has been consistently observed that there is no quantitative change in the collagen content of osteoarthrotic cartilage, qualitative alterations at the molecular level have been demonstrated. Ultrastructural evidence suggests that there is an increase in fibre diameter and that a disruption of the collagen bundles in the surface layers of cartilage is one of the earliest changes in osteoarthrosis (Weiss, 1973). In 1973 Nimni and Deshmukh reported that osteoarthrotic cartilage slices cultured *in vitro* synthesised significant amounts of type I as well as type II collagen. They suggested that this metabolic abnormality would alter the physicochemical properties of the tissue and that this may account for some of the functional defects of osteoarthrotic cartilage. Gay *et al.* (1976) also detected type I collagen in cartilage in the advanced stages of human osteoarthrosis, using specific fluorescent antibodies. Fluorescence was, however, restricted to the small proportion of cells that had undergone cell division and were forming clusters in deep clefts. Reaction due to type II collagen was seen throughout the matrix, suggesting that this was still the major structural component. Other groups have detected a higher solubility of collagen in osteoarthrotic cartilage, but no type I collagen was found in the extract (Herbage *et al.*, 1972). Using gel electrophoresis to compare the acid-soluble collagen of normal and osteoarthrotic cartilage, Fukae *et al.* (1975) could only detect type II collagen. However, on CM-cellulose chromatography both cartilage sources gave peaks in the region where type I collagen peptides elute. Fukae *et al.* (1975) interpreted their results not as a change in collagen type, but possibly as a change in the degree of hydroxylation or glycosylation of the collagen moieties. The findings of Lippiello *et al.* (1977), showing that the hydroxylysine/hydroxyproline ratios remain unchanged in osteoarthrotic cartilage, are also an indication of no major shift in collagen type. A more recent study by Goldwasser *et al.* (1982) concluded that massive deposition of type I collagen occurs only when fibrocartilage is formed. Adam and Deyl (1983) have shown by immunofluorescence the presence of type III collagen, in addition to types I and II, in osteoarthrotic cartilage, and suggest that a shift in gene expression is responsible. Once again, type II and type III collagen were only found in and around the chondrocyte.

It is now well established that the stability of the collagen fibre depends partly on the formation of covalent intermolecular crosslinks. Although this is a potential site at which disruption of the collagen network could occur, the stability of crosslinks was found to be the same in normal and osteoarthrotic cartilage (Herbert *et al.*, 1973). In contrast, joint capsule collagen from osteoarthrotic specimens had a high proportion of labile intermediate crosslinks, suggesting the synthesis of new collagen.

WATER

The amount of water in human articular cartilage gradually decreases with age to approximately 65–75% of the tissue wet weight in adult cartilage. There are also variations in water content through the cartilage depth, with the highest content in the surface layers and the lowest in the deep layers (Bayliss *et al.*, 1983). One of the most striking abnormalities of osteoarthrotic cartilage is the increase in its water content. This has been a consistent finding of numerous studies of fibrillated cartilage samples in the late stages of osteoarthrosis. However, the same phenomenon was found in specimens of non-fibrillated, full-thickness cartilage from osteoarthrotic femoral heads and femoral condyles (Byers *et al.*, 1977; Brocklehurst *et al.*, 1984), suggesting that it may also be one of the earliest biochemical changes.

This is a surprising finding when one considers that the highly hydrophobic proteoglycans, which endow cartilage with its water-imbibing properties, are usually decreasing in fibrillated cartilage. Two independent investigations of this apparent paradox have been carried out. Although both used a similar experimental approach (the exchange of tritiated water between cartilage and medium), different results were obtained by each group. Mankin and Thrasher (1975) noted that osteoarthrotic cartilage 'bound' water more avidly than normal cartilage, and showed that they could duplicate this result by partial extraction of proteoglycan from normal cartilage with 4-molar guanidinium hydrochloride. It was suggested that depletion of proteoglycan exposed binding sites on the collagen molecule, which could hold loosely-bound water to its surface. A possible alternative explanation was that loss of some proteoglycans allowed the remaining aggregates to increase their domain and their affinity for water.

The study carried out by Maroudas and Venn (1977) relied on a physicochemical analysis of the problem. Measurements of equilibrium, partition and diffusion of tritiated water demonstrated that the water in cartilage was entirely free in both normal and degenerate specimens. They suggest that the increase in water content in osteoarthrotic cartilage is due to an impaired collagen network, resulting in a decreased restraining force which fails to oppose the swelling pressure of the proteoglycans. They supported their hypothesis with a simple but elegant experiment, showing that fibrillated cartilage swells when the osmotic stress is increased, whereas normal cartilage does not. Furthermore, swelling was highest in the middle zones where no depletion of proteoglycan had occurred, arguing against a causal relationship between increased hydration and proteoglycan loss. What remains to be established is the cause of the collagen defect.

PROTEOGLYCANS

The most consistent biochemical change observed in osteoarthrotic articular cartilage is a loss of proteoglycan. This was originally seen histochemically as a loss of metachromatic staining with basic dyes in the extracellular matrix. Since then, many investigators have reported a decrease in one or more of the glycosaminoglycans in diseased cartilage. Mankin et al. (1971) have also established that the decrease is directly proportional to the severity of the lesion in samples obtained from resected femoral heads, and Byers et al. (1977) came to the same conclusion when comparing early and late osteoarthrotic lesions.

More extensive studies have shown that the changes in proteoglycan composition are not uniform. This may be the result of differences in tissue sampling and variations in the extent of the lesion within any joint. Furthermore, little attention has been paid to errors that will arise when comparisons are made between full-thickness, normal cartilage and thinner, diseased cartilage (i.e. the comparison is only correct if made between corresponding zones through the cartilage depth). Nevertheless one of the most consistent findings is a decrease in the proportion of keratan sulphate relative to chrondroitin sulphate (Mankin and Lippiello, 1971; Ali and Bayliss, 1974; Suzuki et al., 1978; Sweet et al., 1977). A significant increase in the proportion of chondroitin 4-sulphate in pathological specimens was also found by Mankin and Lippiello (1971), but Hjertquist and Lemperg (1972) reported that the proportions of these two

isomers were unchanged. Bollet and Nance (1966) have also shown a decrease in the average chain length of chondroitin sulphate, a finding subsequently confirmed by Hjertquist and Wasteson (1972). The concentration of hyaluronic acid, the polysaccharide vital for aggregation of proteoglycans and their immobilisation in cartilage matrix, is also decreased in osteoarthrotic specimens (Thonar et al., 1978). This important finding was however based on analysis of only two samples and has not been confirmed.

The relationship between these changes in tissue chemistry and altered macromolecular structure has not been systematically investigated and is still unclear. Sweet et al. (1977) have suggested that the proteoglycans purified from osteoarthrotic cartilage are carbohydrate deficient and are more soluble. A decreased content of keratan sulphate and protein was also noted for the proteoglycans extracted from cartilage of resected femoral heads (Bayliss and Ali, 1978a; Bayliss and Venn, 1980), whereas a similar study of femoral condyles did not show these changes (Brocklehurst et al., 1984). Preliminary results suggest that the altered composition results from a decreased content of low molecular weight proteoglycan that is characteristic of adult cartilage (Bayliss and Venn, 1980; Bayliss et al., 1983).

An abnormality in aggregation, either as a defect in link-protein or the hyaluronic acid-binding region of the proteoglycan molecule, has often been suggested as one route by which proteoglycans are lost from the tissue. However, there is little evidence for this hypothesis in human osteoarthrotic cartilage. Ryu et al. (1982) have shown that link-proteins from normal and diseased cartilage are chemically and functionally identical. Furthermore, the proteoglycans remaining in osteoarthrotic cartilage from the femoral head and femoral condyle aggregate to the same extent as those from normal cartilage (Bayliss and Venn, 1980; Brocklehurst et al., 1984). However, Mort et al. (1983) have recently demonstrated a fragmentation of the link-proteins with increasing age in normal human cartilage and have suggested that this may have some bearing on aggregate stability.

METABOLIC CHANGES

The obvious loss of proteoglycan from osteoarthrotic cartilage has prompted many investigations of the chondrocytes' ability to repair the depleted matrix. This in turn has resulted in one of the most controversial issues concerning the biochemistry of osteoarthrosis. In 1960, Collins and McElligott used autoradiography to show that osteoarthrotic cartilage was metabolically more active than normal cartilage, as measured by the incorporation of $^{35}SO_4$.

Since then many other investigators have supported the finding that osteoarthrotic cartilage has an increased rate of proteoglycan synthesis (Mankin et al., 1971; Jacoby and Jayson, 1976; Thompson and Oegema, 1979; Mitrovic et al., 1981).

However, other groups do not agree with these findings and suggest that there is no difference, or even a slight decrease, in the rate of synthesis of osteoarthrotic cartilage compared with normal (McKenzie et al., 1977; Maroudas, 1975; Byers et al., 1977; Brocklehurst et al., 1984). From the published data, it is difficult to account for this difference in results. Many factors could be responsible, since the techniques used are not identical and tissue sampling is probably not uniform. Some progress could be made towards explaining the data of different laboratories if results were expressed in the same units (i.e. mmoles of sulphate incorporated per hour per gram of tissue). This at least would show whether the normal cartilage used by different groups was similar in activity.

Extensive investigations by Mankin and colleagues have shown that, regardless of whether $^{35}SO_4$ or ^{3}H-glucosamine is used as a precursor, synthesis rates are increased to parallel the severity of the disease process (Mankin et al., 1981). Similar results were obtained when isolated proteoglycans were studied after labelling with $^{35}SO_4$, ^{3}H-glucosamine and ^{3}H-leucine. All the components of proteoglycan aggregate (subunit, hyaluronic acid and link-protein) were labelled but the relative rate of synthesis of proteoglycan subunit was greater in the osteoarthrotic cartilage. Although the total ^{3}H-glucosamine incorporation was increased, the ratio of incorporation into glucosamine and galactosamine was the same in normal and osteoarthrotic cartilage, suggesting that the product was probably similar in composition.

A more recent study from the same laboratory has shown that chondrocytes isolated from osteoarthrotic cartilage retain their increased synthesis rate compared to normal chondrocytes (Teshima et al., 1983). This finding is important because it suggests that feedback from the proteoglycan-depleted matrix is not the only factor stimulating synthesis. However, it would be interesting to know how long the diseased cells retain this property.

Whether proteoglycan synthesis is elevated or not, the times calculated for turnover, 300–600 days in adult cartilage (Maroudas, 1975), suggest that repair of a progressive lesion would not be very effective. If, however, there are proteoglycan pools that have a high turnover, focal repair might be possible. The same reasoning applies to the metabolism of collagen. Here again the turnover time is estimated to be in the order of 500 years (Maroudas, 1975); the elevated synthesis rates observed by Lippiello et al. (1977) would therefore have little effect.

ENZYMES

The dramatic effect of proteolytic enzymes on the degradation of cartilage in vivo (Thomas, 1956) and of similar agents in producing osteoarthrosis in animals has led to the suggestion that there may be potent enzymes present in cartilage which bring about its rapid breakdown. The most effective way of disrupting

the proteoglycan aggregate structure would be to degrade the hyaluronic acid. However, there is no direct evidence of hyaluronidase activity in articular cartilage (Bollet, 1967), although Leaback (1974) has suggested that this could happen through the combined action of endo- and exoglycosidases. Systematic investigations of the endogenous enzymes present in cartilage that may cause degradation of the matrix from within have been made in several laboratories (Ali, 1964; Chrisman, 1969; Dingle, 1973; Howell and Bollet, 1973) and have centred on the lysosomal acid proteinases. Which of these enzymes (if any) play a significant role in cartilage degeneration, and at what stage of the disease process they are involved, is still not clear. A significant increase in acid phosphatase, which is a general marker for lysosomal activity, has been demonstrated in osteoarthrotic cartilage (Ali and Bayliss, 1974). The degree of increase has also been shown to be directly proportional to the severity of the lesion (Ehrlich et al., 1973). These results supported the hypothesis that the enzyme changes were the result of an increase in the lysosome content of the tissue. In early studies of human osteoarthrosis considerable emphasis was placed on a specific proteinase, cathepsin D, as the enzyme most likely to cause cartilage degradation. Thus, Ali and Evans (1973) presented evidence for a raised level of cathepsin D in cartilage

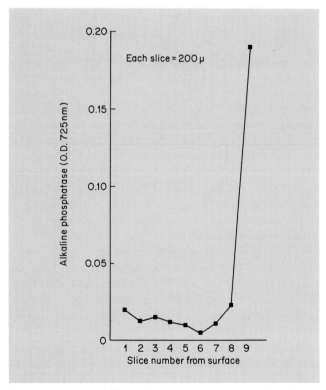

Fig. 1. Distribution of alkaline phosphatase (measured by the hydrolysis of sodium beta-glycerophosphate) through the depth of adult human articular cartilage (femoral head). Histochemical localisation of alkaline phosphatase (using naphthol AS-BI phosphate as substrate) in 10 μm section of human articular cartilage incubated for 10 minutes.

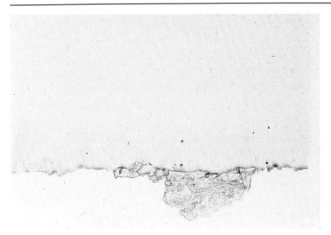

Fig. 2. Adult cartilage (56 years). Only a few cells show enzyme activity. (× 38)

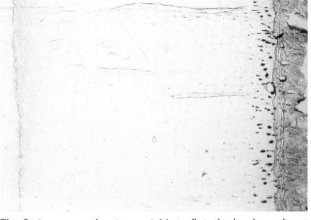

Fig. 3. Immature cartilage (10 years). Most cells in the deep layer adjacent to the subchondral bone are active. (× 24)

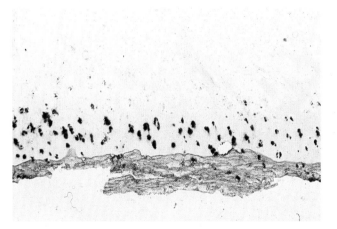

Fig. 4. Osteoarthrotic cartilage (60 years). Most cells in the deep layer are very active. (× 38)

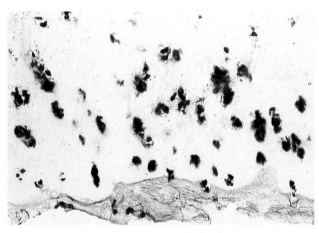

Fig. 5. Higher power view of active cells in the deep layer. (× 95)

from resected femoral heads, both on a wet weight and a DNA basis. More important was their observation of a femoral head from an amputated specimen, the zenith of which showed the first signs of fraying and tissue granulation. Here again, cathepsin D activity was high when compared with the normal surrounding cartilage. At the same time, Sapolsky et al. (1973) showed that extracts of ulcerated cartilage from patients with primary osteoarthrosis contained two to three times more cathepsin D-type enzyme activity than control specimens. There is now considerable evidence that cathepsin D has no action at neutral pH, and that more acid pH conditions would have to prevail locally for it to effect significant degradation of the proteoglycans (Woessner, 1973; Sapolsky et al., 1974). Dingle et al. (1972), working with human articular cartilage, showed that inhibition of autolysis with pepstatin (a potent inhibitor of cathepsin D) still resulted in activity at pH 6·0 which amounted to 20% of that attributable to cathepsin D at pH 5·0. The pH 6·0 activity was enhanced by EDTA and by dithiothreitol, but inhibited by iodoacetate and other thiolenzyme inhibitors—which was con-

sistent with cathepsin B-like activity. Using a chromogenic substrate for cathepsin B, Bayliss and Ali (1978b) confirmed the presence of this enzyme in human cartilage and its elevated activity in osteoarthrotic cartilage.

More recently, Sapolsky et al. (1976) and Sapolsky and Howell (1982) have isolated a neutral metalloproteinase from human patella cartilage. The enzyme degraded proteoglycan subunit and aggregate at neutral pH and may, therefore, play a more significant role in the turnover of macromolecules in the extracellular matrix. Furthermore, the role of synovial enzymes in cartilage breakdown in osteoarthrosis has been studied by Gedikoglu et al. (1985), who found high levels of proteinase activity in non-rheumatoid synovium; but the significance of these findings is not clear. The enzymic degradation of collagen has received little attention in the past because the collagen content is unchanged even in cartilage samples severely depleted of proteoglycan. However, minor changes in the collagen network could influence the swelling observed in the middle zones of osteoarthrotic cartilage (Maroudas, 1976). Recent studies by

Ehrlich *et al.* (1978) have shown the presence of collagenase in the culture fluid of osteoarthrotic cartilage, the enzyme activity increasing with the severity of the lesion.

Apart from the cartilage destruction that is characteristic of osteoarthrosis, the most striking feature of the advanced specimens is the extensive remodelling that occurs. This is most readily recognised by the development of marginal osteophytes, but laying down of new bone in the areas of active cartilage erosion is also evident. Observations by Johnson (1962) led him to the idea of continuous remodelling of subchondral bone as a general concept. In a study of adult human patellae, Green *et al.* (1970) concluded that there is continuous growth activity in the osteochondral region during adult life. From their biochemical and enzymic analyses of human osteoarthrotic cartilage, Ali and Evans (1973) postulated a calcification abnormality in diseased tissue as one aetiological factor. Electron-microscopy of diseased cartilage demonstrated amorphous and crystalline mineral deposits in cartilage matrix (Ali and Bayliss, 1974; Ali and Wisby, 1975). Ultrastructural examination of normal articular cartilage also confirmed that the tissue contained matrix vesicles similar to those involved in the initial stages of mineralisation of growth cartilage. This high level of alkaline phosphatase in the vesicles enabled a quantitative assessment of normal and diseased cartilage to be carried out. A comparative study demonstrated that there was a significant elevation of alkaline phosphatase in the diseased tissue (Ali and Evans, 1973; Ali and Bayliss, 1974). Figure 1 shows that in normal cartilage the enzyme is confined to the deepest level near the tide-mark region. Enzyme histochemical analysis of tissue sections confirmed this finding (Fig. 2) and also demonstrated the higher levels of enzyme found in immature cartilage where growth is still occurring (Fig. 3). In osteoarthrotic cartilage, enzyme activity is much higher, as shown by an increased deposition of diazo-dye in and around the chondrocytes (Figs 4 and 5). It is also more prevalent in the middle zones of the tissue, in agreement with the ultrastructural evidence described by Ali (1978).

These studies led Ali (1978) to propose that it might be appropriate to regard articular cartilage (especially near the osteochondral junction) as latent growth plate that can revert to a growth phase under various pathological conditions. Remodelling of the osteochondral junction may alter the mechanical properties of the remaining layers of cartilage, which may then become more susceptible to degradation by normal wear processes, as indicated by Johnson (1962).

REFERENCES

ADAM, M. and DEYL, Z. (1983) Altered expression of collagen phenotype in osteoarthrosis. *Clin. Chim. Acta* **133**, 25–32.

ALI, S.Y. (1964) The degradation of cartilage matrix by an intra cellular protease. *Biochem. J.* **93**, 611–618.

ALI, S.Y. (1978) New knowledge of osteoarthrosis. In: *Diseases of Connective Tissue*, D.L. Gardner (Ed.), pp. 191–199. Royal College of Pathologists, London.

ALI, S.Y. and BAYLISS, M.T. (1974) Enzymic changes in human osteoarthrotic cartilage. In: *Normal and Osteoarthrotic Articular Cartilage*, S.Y. Ali *et al.* (Eds), pp. 189–202. Institute of Orthopaedics, London.

ALI, S.Y. and EVANS, L. (1973) Enzymic degradation of cartilage in osteoarthritis. *Fed. Proc.* **32**, 1494–1498.

ALI, S.Y. and WISBY, A. (1975) Ultrastructural aspects of normal and osteoarthrotic cartilage. *Ann. Rheum. Dis.* **34** (Suppl. 2), 21–23.

BAYLISS, M.T. and ALI, S.Y. (1978a) Studies on cathepsin B in human articular cartilage. *Biochem. J.* **171**, 149–154.

BAYLISS, M.T. and ALI, S.Y. (1978b) Isolation of proteoglycans from human articular cartilage. *Biochem. J.* **169**, 123–132.

BAYLISS, M.T. and VENN, M. (1980) Chemistry of human articular cartilage. In: *Studies in Joint Disease*, A. Maroudas and E.J. Holborrow (Eds), Vol. 1, pp. 2–58. Pitman Medical, London.

BAYLISS, M.T., VENN, M., MAROUDAS, A. and ALI, S.Y. (1983) Structure of proteoglycans from different layers of human articular cartilage. *Biochem. J.* **209**, 387–400.

BOLLET, A.J. (1967) Connective tissue polysaccharide metabolism and pathogenesis of osteoarthritis. *Adv. Intern. Med.* **13**, 33–60.

BOLLET, A.J. and NANCE, J.L. (1966) Biochemical findings in normal and osteoarthritic articular cartilage. II. Chondroitin sulfate concentration and chain length, water, and ash content. *J. Clin. Invest.* **45**, 1170–1177.

BROCKLEHURST, R., BAYLISS, M.T., MAROUDAS, A., COYSH, H.L., FREEMAN, M.A.R., REVELL, P.A. and ALI, S.Y. (1984) The composition of normal and osteoarthritic articular cartilage from human knee joints: with special reference to unicompartmental replacement and osteotomy of the knee. *J. Bone Joint Surg.* **66**A, 95–106.

BYERS, P.D., MAROUDAS, A., OZTOP, F., STOCKWELL, R.A. and VENN, M.F. (1977) Histological and biochemical studies on cartilage from osteoarthrotic femoral heads with special reference to surface characteristics. *Connect. Tissue Res.* **5**, 41–49.

CHRISMAN, O.D. (1969) Biochemical aspects of degenerative joint disease. *Clin. Orthop.* **64**, 77–86.

COLLINS, D.H. (1949) *The Pathology of Articular and Spinal Disease.* E. Arnold, London.

COLLINS, D.H. and McELLIGOTT, T.F. (1960) Sulphate uptake by chondrocytes in relation to histological changes in osteoarthritic human articular cartilage. *Ann. Rheum. Dis.* **19**, 318–322.

DINGLE, J.T. (1973) The role of lysosomal enzymes in skeletal tissues. *J. Bone Joint Surg.* **55**B, 87–95.

DINGLE, J.T., BARRETT, A.J., POOLE, A.R. and STOVIN, P. (1972) Inhibition by pepstatin of human cartilage degradation. *Biochem. J.* **127**, 443–444.

EHRLICH, M.G., HOULE, P.A., VIGLIANI, G. and MANKIN, H.J. (1978)

Correlation between articular cartilage collagenase activity and osteoarthritis. *Arthritis Rheum.* **21**, 761–766.

EHRLICH, M.G., MANKIN, M.G. and TREADWELL, B.V. (1973) Acid hydrolase activity in osteoarthritic and normal human cartilage. *J. Bone Joint Surg.* **55**A, 1068–1076.

FUKAE, M., MECHANIC, G.L., ADAMY, L. and SCHWARTZ, E.R. (1975) Chromatographically different type II collagens from human normal and osteoarthritic cartilage. *Biochem. Biophys. Res. Commun.* **69**, 1575–1580.

GAY, S., MÜLLER, P.K., LEMMEN, C., REMBERGER, K., MATZEN, K. and KUHN, K. (1976) Immunohistological study on collagen in cartilage-bone metamorphoses and degenerative arthritis. *Klin. Wochenschr.* **54**, 969–976.

GEDIKOGLU, O., BAYLISS, M.T., ALI, S.Y. and TUNCER, I. (1985) Biochemical and histological changes in osteoarthritic synovial membrane. *Ann. Rheum. Dis.* (in press).

GOLDWASSER, M., ASTLEY, T., VAN DER REST, M. and GLORIEUX, F.H. (1982) Analysis of the type of collagen present in osteoarthritic human cartilage. *Clin. Orthop. Rel. Res.* **167**, 296–302.

GREEN, W.T., MARTIN, G.N., EANES, E.D. and SOKOLOFF, L. (1970) Microradiographic study of the calcified layer of articular cartilage. *Arch. Pathol.* **90**, 151–158.

HERBAGE, D., HUC, A., CHABRAND, D. and CHAPUY, M.C. (1972) Physicochemical study of articular cartilage from healthy osteoarthritic human hips. Orientation and thermal stability of collagen fibres. *Biochim. Biophys. Acta* **271**, 339–346.

HERBERT, C., JAYSON, M.I. and BAILEY, A.J. (1973) Joint capsule collagen in osteoarthrosis. *Ann. Rheum. Dis.* **32**, 510–514.

HJERTQUIST, S.O. and LEMPERG, R.C. (1972) Identification and concentration of the glycosaminoglycans of human articular cartilage in relation to age and osteoarthritis. *Calcif. Tiss. Res.* **10**, 223–237.

HJERTQUIST, S.O. and WASTESON, A. (1972) The molecular weight of chondroitin sulphate from human articular cartilage. *Calcif. Tiss. Res.* **10**, 31–37.

HOWELL, D.S. and BOLLET, A.J. (1973) Workshop on osteoarthrosis. *Fed. Proc.* **32**, 1457–1506.

JACOBY, R.K. and JAYSON, M.I.V. (1976) The organ culture of adult human articular cartilage from patients with osteoarthrosis. *Rheumatol. Rehabil.* **15**, 116–122.

JOHNSON, L.C. (1962) Joint remodelling as a basis for osteoarthritis. *J. Am. Vet. Med. Assoc.* **141**, 1237–1241.

LEABACK, D.H. (1974) Studies on some glycosidases from the chondrocytes of articular cartilage and from certain other cells and tissues. In: *Normal and Osteoarthrotic Articular Cartilage*, S.Y. Ali *et al.* (Eds), pp. 73–83. Institute of Orthopaedics, London.

LIPPIELLO, L., HALL, D. and MANKIN, H.J. (1977) Collagen synthesis in normal and osteoarthritic human cartilage. *J. Clin. Invest.* **59**, 593–600.

McKENZIE, L.S., HORSBURGH, B.A., GHOSH, P. and TAYLOR, T.K.F.

(1977) Sulphated glycosaminoglycan synthesis in normal and osteoarthritic hip cartilage. *Ann. Rheum. Dis.* **36**, 369–373.

MANKIN, H.J., DORFMAN, H., LIPPIELLO, L. and ZARINS, A. (1971) Biochemical and metabolic abnormalities in articular cartilage from osteoarthritic human hips. II. Correlation of morphology with biochemical and metabolic data. *J. Bone Joint Surg.* **53**A, 523–537.

MANKIN, H.J., JOHNSON, M.E. and LIPPIELLO, L. (1981) Biochemical and metabolic abnormalities in articular cartilage from osteoarthritic human hips. III. Distribution and metabolism of amino sugar-containing macromolecules. *J. Bone Joint Surg.* **63**A, 131–139.

MANKIN, H.J. and LIPPIELLO, L. (1971) The glycosaminoglycans of normal and arthritic cartilage. *J. Clin. Invest.* **50**, 1712–1719.

MANKIN, H.J. and THRASHER, A.Z. (1975) Water content and binding in normal and osteoarthritic human cartilage. *J. Bone Joint Surg.* **57**A, 76–79.

MAROUDAS, A. (1975) Glycosaminoglycan turnover in articular cartilage. *Philos. Trans. R. Soc. Lond.* [Biol.] **271**, 293–313.

MAROUDAS, A. (1976) Balance between swelling pressure and collagen tension in normal and degenerate cartilage. *Nature* **260**, 214–216.

MAROUDAS, A. and VENN, M. (1977) Chemical composition and swelling of normal and osteoarthrotic femoral head cartilage. II. Swelling. *Ann. Rheum. Dis.* **36**, 399–406.

MITROVIC, D., GRUSON, M., DEMIGNON, J., MERCIER, P., APRILE, F. and DeSEZE, S. (1981) Metabolism of human femoral head cartilage in osteoarthrosis and subcapital fracture. *Ann. Rheum. Dis.* **40**, 18–26.

MORT, J.S., POOLE, A.R. and ROUGHLEY, P.J. (1983) Age-related changes in the structure of proteoglycan link proteins present in normal human articular cartilage. *Biochem. J.* **214**, 269–272.

NIMNI, M. and DESHMUKH, K. (1973) Differences in collagen metabolism between normal and osteoarthrotic human articular cartilage. *Science* **181**, 751–752.

RYU, J., TOWLE, C.A. and TREADWELL, B.V. (1982) Characterisation of human articular cartilage link proteins from normal and osteoarthritic cartilage. *Ann. Rheum. Dis.* **41**, 164–167.

SAPOLSKY, A.I., ALTMAN, R.D. and HOWELL, D.S. (1973) Cathepsin D activity in normal and osteoarthrotic human cartilage. *Fed. Proc.* **32**, 1489–1493.

SAPOLSKY, A.I. and HOWELL, D.S. (1982) Further characterisation of a neutral metalloprotease isolated from human articular cartilage. *Arthritis Rheum.* **25**, 981–988.

SAPOLSKY, A.I., HOWELL, D.S. and WOESSNER, J.F. (1974) Neutral proteases and cathepsin D in human articular cartilage. *J. Clin. Invest.* **53**, 1044–1053.

SAPOLSKY, A.I., KEISER, H., HOWELL, D.S. and WOESSNER, J.F. Jr (1976) Metalloproteases of human articular cartilage that digest cartilage proteoglycan at neutral and acid pH. *J. Clin. Invest.* **58**, 1030–1041.

SUZUKI, M., BOERSMA, A., DEGAND, P. and BISERTE, G. (1978)

55

Etude biochimique comparative des glycosaminoglycannes peptides du cartilage articulaire de la tête femorale humaine normale et arthrosique. *Clin. Chim. Acta* **87**, 229–238.

SWEET, M.B., THONAR, J., IMMELMAN, A.R. and SOLOMON, L. (1977) Biochemical changes in progressive osteoarthrosis. *Ann. Rheum. Dis.* **36**, 387–398.

TESHIMA, R., TREADWELL, B.V., TREHAN, C.A. and MANKIN, H.A. (1983) Comparative rates of proteoglycan synthesis and size of proteoglycans in normal and osteoarthrotic chondrocytes. *Arthritis Rheum.* **26**, 1225–1230.

THOMAS, L. (1956) Reversible collapse of rabbit ears after intravenous papain and prevention of recovery by cortisone.

J. Exp. Med. **104**, 245–252.

THOMPSON, R.C. and OEGEMA, T.R. (1979) Synthesis of proteoglycans in osteoarthritic human articular cartilage. *J. Bone Joint Surg.* **61**A, 407–417.

THONAR, E.J.-M.A., SWEET, M.B.E., IMMELMAN, A.R. and LYONS, G. (1978) Hyaluronate in articular cartilage. Age-related changes. *Calcif. Tiss. Res.* **26**, 19–21.

WEISS, C. (1973) Ultrastructural characteristics of osteoarthritis. *Fed. Proc.* **32**, 1459–1466.

WOESSNER, J.F. (1973) Purification of cathepsin D from cartilage and uterus and its action on the protein–polysaccharide complex of cartilage. *J. Biol. Chem.* **248**, 1634–1642.

Chapter 4

On the Pathogenesis of Canine Osteoarthritis

GEORGE LUST and NANCY B. WURSTER

James A. Baker Institute for Animal Health, New York State College of Veterinary Medicine,
Cornell University, Ithaca, New York, USA

SUMMARY

Hip dysplasia in labrador retrievers is an instructive model for the study of early changes in human osteoarthritis (OA). These include localised cartilage fibrillation, swelling of the round ligament, and synovitis with effusion occurring at the same time as articular cartilage degeneration and preceding signs of subluxation of the femoral head.

The first change observed is abrasion of the protective layer of amorphous material covering the cartilage surface, followed by exposure of the underlying collagen and loosening of their bundles. Also, the proportion of synovial cell types change, suggesting incipient synovial inflammation at an earlier stage than previously recognised in the course of OA. No association with developmental abnormalities in hip conformation has yet been demonstrated, but the possibility remains.

In dysplasia-prone dogs, similar events occur in other joints. Those destined to become the seat of OA can be identified early by the biochemical and physiological changes they show. Collagen is synthesised and deposited more slowly in fibrillated areas of cartilage than in adjacent, 'unaffected' areas and the characteristic banding pattern is then lost. Fibronectin levels in synovial fluid (but not plasma) are raised in this model of OA, probably indicating cartilage destruction. Other materials also accumulate, but these have not yet been characterised.

The osteoarthritis (degenerative joint disease, osteoarthrosis) which occurs in conjunction with canine hip dysplasia resembles the human disease, coxarthrosis. It is not confined to the hip joints in dogs, as similar changes also occur in the knee and shoulder joints of some dysplasia-prone animals.

The justified concern regarding the general relevance of animal models to human disease includes hip dysplasia and osteoarthritis in labrador retriever dogs. Nevertheless, there are remarkable parallels between the canine and human joint diseases and compelling reasons for selecting the canine disorder as a model for study. Hip dysplasia in dogs occurs spontaneously and evolves slowly; selective breeding has produced animals with enhanced susceptibility. At the morphological and biochemical level, the tissues from diseased canine and human joints show striking similarities (Adams and Billingham, 1982). These considerations and the results described in the following sections of this paper encourage the belief that hip dysplasia in labrador retrievers provides an instructive model of early events in the human osteoarthritic process.

MORPHOLOGY OF CARTILAGE AND SYNOVIUM

Among the early intra-articular alterations observed in dysplastic hip joints were focal areas of fibrillated cartilage at a topologically constant site on the femoral head. Proliferative synovitis was also observed. Inflammation of the synovium correlated with increased synovial fluid volume and round ligament volume in the affected joint (Lust and Summers, 1981). It is not known whether the observed changes are causally related. However, the increase in synovial fluid volume coincided with histological and histochemical evidence of articular cartilage degeneration, and preceded the development of subluxation of the femoral head as detected by clinical or radiographic examination of the joint (Table I). Thus, the changes in articular cartilage were shown to be an early change in joints destined to become the seat of the osteoarthritic process.

The volume of synovial fluid in the disease-free hip joints ranged from 0·05–0·4 ml; shoulder joints contained 0·1–0·5 ml. In the early disease, joints with fibrillated cartilage contained fluid volumes of significantly greater volume (hips 0·5–10·0 ml; shoulders 0·6–1·6 ml) (Lust et al., 1980; Lust and Summers, 1981; Olsewski et al., 1983). The protein concentration and the osmolality of the synovial fluids of osteoarthritic joints were increased significantly compared to synovial fluid from disease-free joints (Olsewski et al., 1983). Data illustrating this are presented in Table I. Values of fluids from hip and shoulder joints were combined. The mechanism causing increased volumes of synovial fluid to accumulate is not yet known.

Electron microscopic studies disclosed a relationship between cartilage degeneration and synovial changes in the hip joints of the experimental dogs early in the course of the disease (Greisen et al., 1982). In joints with normal cartilage, i.e. no surface roughening (fibrillation) and normal distribution of chondrocytes and proteoglycans, the synovium contained approximately 33% type A and 64% type B cells, with only small numbers of necrotic and infiltrating cells. The earliest signs of injury to the cartilage were focal defects in the layer of amorphous material covering the cartilage surface. With the loss of this protective layer, collagen fibrils and bundles became exposed and loosened. Crystals were not observed in fibrillated

Table I. Protein concentration and osmolality of synovial fluids from disease-free and osteoarthritic joints

Type of joint	Protein (g/dl)	Osmolality (mOs/kg)
Disease-free joints	(22) 1·55 ± 0·49	(32) 260 ± 22
Osteoarthritic joints	(50) 2·21 ± 0·62	(44) 311 ± 34

Data as means and s.d. Numbers in parentheses were number of samples tested. Protein by Biuret method; osmolality by vapour pressure osmometer at room temperature. Range of serum protein concentration of dogs was 5·70–7·40 g/dl; range of serum osmolality of dogs was 250–320 mOs/kg. Mean protein concentration and mean osmolality of synovial fluids from disease-free joints differed significantly ($P < 0.05$) from osteoarthritic fluids. Disease-free joints contained low volumes of synovial fluid and normal cartilage; osteoarthritic joints contained increased fluid volumes and fibrillated or degenerated cartilage (Olsewski et al., 1983).

cartilage. When early focal defects of the cartilage surface were present the percentage of type A cells in synovium decreased from 33% to 15% ($P < 0.05$) and necrotic cells and cells of uncertain type increased from less than 5% to about 16%, whereas the percentage of type B cells remained unchanged. Proliferation of cells occurred in the intimal layer in synovitis, though the proportional distribution of A and B cells described above was maintained in more advanced stages of degenerative joint disease. Thus, quantitative ultrastructural studies revealed changes in synoviocyte distribution which we concluded preceded overt synovial inflammation as evaluated by light microscopy.

These observations have implications for the development of osteoarthritis in disease-prone dogs, because the changes occurred early in the disease. They suggest that abrasion of the cartilage surface is a critical event. Cell proliferation and inflammatory processes in the synovium also seem to be involved earlier in the progression of osteoarthritis than has been reported. It seems plausible to reason that synovitis occurs in response to cartilage products that are released from the injured cartilage.

Possible developmental abnormalities of the opposing faces in the hip joint were considered as factors favouring the expression of hip dysplasia, e.g. reduction in the depth of the acetabulum (assessed on radiograph), the degree of inclination of the femoral head, and anteversion of the femoral head due to abnormal torsion or twisting of the femur. But measurements performed on anatomical specimens from 'high-risk' dogs and disease-free subjects failed to reveal significant differences in these parameters (Lust et al., unpublished results). Although these studies proved unrewarding, subtle but as yet unrecognised changes in conformation of the hip joint must still be considered as pathogenic factors. For example, precise physical measurements of the acetabulum might reveal subtle changes that could not be detected by radiographic examination of the hip joint.

Multi-joint involvement

Cartilage degeneration and associated changes in the joint were not restricted to the hip joints of young dogs. The shoulder and knee joints were also affected in many dogs of our disease-prone line (Olsewski et al., 1983). Abnormalities also occurred in elbow and lumbar vertebral joints in older dogs, but these joints have not yet been examined in detail. Cartilage fibrillation and/or concomitants of osteoarthritis, such as a significant increase in synovial fluid volume (Table I) and histological evidence of synovial membrane inflammation, were observed frequently in the shoulder and knee joints as well as in the hip joints of disease-prone young dogs. Focal areas of fibrillated cartilage were observed on the femoral head (Fig. 1), on the medial tibial plateau (and sometimes the lateral plateau also), and on the humeral head. All cartilage lesions appeared velvety grey

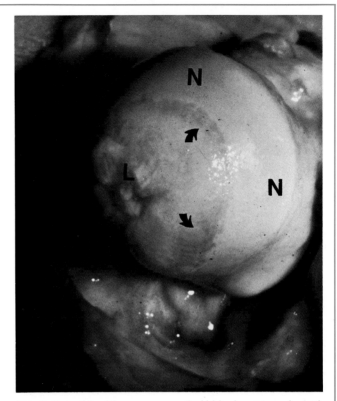

Fig. 1. Femoral head from a seven-month-old labrador retriever dog with bilateral displacement of femoral heads, i.e. hip dysplasia. Hip joint had increased synovial fluid volume, synovitis, enlarged ligament and fibrillated, eroded articular cartilage. Arrows point to region of degenerated cartilage; N = 'normal', less affected adjacent articular cartilage; L = ligament.

after application of carbon black (Indian ink), and histochemical analysis revealed surface fibrillation and loss of proteoglycans. Water content was reproducibly increased by about 5% in the fibrillated areas when compared to the surrounding cartilage of the same joint surface and to cartilage of disease-free joints. Collagen deposition was reduced, as quantified by radio-labelled hydroxyproline accumulation in the matrix (to be described in full detail below). A similar reduction of collagen deposition was documented in the fibrillated cartilage from femoral heads of osteoarthritic hip joints. Although unambiguous signs of cartilage fibrillation and erosion were observed frequently in many joints examined at necropsy, we have been unable to determine whether hip joint dysplasia is simply the most conspicuous manifestation of a disease affecting multiple joints, or whether the observed cartilage fibrillation and joint effusions in other joints are biochemical sequelae of the hip abnormality. The biomechanical hypothesis is not supported by the observation that in some dogs the stifle and/or shoulder joints revealed cartilage degeneration, but hip joints appeared normal (Olsewski et al., 1983). We have not determined whether the early changes observed in the shoulder and knee joints of young dogs would have resulted ultimately in other changes characteristic of osteoarthritis. This is likely because these joints and the hip joints are frequently sites of clinical osteoarthritis in older dogs (Pedersen and Pool, 1978).

The data described above represent X-ray and pathological observations in young and old dogs (Olsewski *et al.*, 1983). More importantly, early biochemical changes were identified in the joints that apparently are destined to be the seat of frank osteoarthritis as animals get older. The observed multiple joint involvement in dogs was similar to that reported by several groups for some types of polyarthritis in humans (Cooke *et al.*, 1980; Huskisson *et al.*, 1979; Kellgren and Moore, 1952; Yazici *et al.*, 1975).

CARTILAGE COLLAGEN METABOLISM

Type of collagen

Normally type II collagen is formed in cartilage. But in studies undertaken with cartilage from human subjects with advanced osteoarthritis, evidence for a switch to type I synthesis was reported (Nimni and Deshmukh, 1973). Other investigators failed to detect type I collagen in experimentally induced disease in animals (Eyre *et al.*, 1980; Floman *et al.*, 1980).

The collagen in the degenerated cartilage from osteoarthritic canine joints was characterised by examining cartilage directly and comparing it with cartilage which had been labelled with ^{14}C-proline *in vitro* (Hui-Chou and Lust, 1982). Analysis employed sodium dodecylsulphate-polyacrylamide gel electrophoresis of ^{14}C-labelled collagen, and of ^{14}C-peptides which had been cleaved by cyanogen bromide, and by amino-acid analysis of hydrolysates of whole cartilage samples (degenerated control). Cartilage collagen was purified by fractional precipitation. Purified preparations were used to quantify the content of hydroxyproline and hydroxylysine; the ratio of hydroxyproline to hydroxylysine has been used to characterise collagen types. Data from the biochemical analyses revealed that type II collagen was the radio-labelled product in all samples of degenerative cartilage and was the only collagen detected in chemical tests in the degenerative cartilage of osteoarthritic canine joints. The results supported the concept that chondrocytes in degenerated cartilage of osteoarthritic canine joints did not switch their collagen phenotype but continued to synthesise only type II collagen. We concluded that cartilage degeneration in osteoarthritic joints of dogs proceeded without a change in collagen phenotype (Hui-Chou and Lust, 1982).

Collagen deposition into the matrix

Our studies indicated that the rate of collagen synthesis and the deposition of newly made collagen into the matrix was reduced in the fibrillated areas of cartilage (Wurster *et al.*, 1982). The

adjacent 'unaffected' cartilage of the same joint (Fig. 1) was normal in its water content, cellularity, proteoglycan, hydroxyproline, and fibronectin content, collagenolytic enzyme activity, and in synthesis and deposition of collagen (Lust *et al.*, 1972; Wurster *et al.*, 1982; Wurster and Lust, 1982). This was shown to be true even in joints with markedly increased synovial fluid volume and histologically documented synovitis. Recently it has been reported that proteoglycan, DNA and protein synthesis did not increase in parallel with degenerative cartilage changes either in human (Byers *et al.*, 1977) or in experimental (Moskowitz *et al.*, 1981) forms of osteoarthritis.

Factors released from the synovial membrane during synovitis might be expected to act as mediators of a general cartilage effect. However, this hypothesis is difficult to reconcile with the discrete, focal nature of cartilage ulceration on affected joint surfaces. The focal areas of fibrillation occur in topologically constant regions of the femoral head, the humeral head, and the medial tibial plateau of affected joints. Thus, there is a major problem in explaining why collagen and proteoglycans are initially depleted in the focal region where the cartilage surface becomes fibrillated. In more advanced disease the entire cartilage surface may be abnormal.

Collagen metabolism in the fibrillated cartilage from dogs with degenerative joint disease was compared with that in the adjacent 'normal' cartilage of the same joint surface (Wurster *et al.*, 1982). The deposition of collagen into the cartilage *in vitro* was significantly decreased ($P < 0.05$) in the early and the advanced stages of cartilage degeneration. The deposition of collagen into cartilage *in vivo* was also reduced in the fibrillated cartilage of two dogs with degenerative joint disease. Gel electrophoretic analysis revealed that degenerated cartilage contained less alpha$_1$ collagen chains, but increased amounts of larger proteins. In other analyses, degenerated cartilage contained more water, increased amounts of fibronectin, greater collagenolytic enzyme activity and fewer chondrocytes.

In vitro studies of collagen biosynthesis have been substantiated by examining the *in vivo* conversion of intravenously injected ^{3}H-proline to ^{3}H-hydroxyproline in the cartilage of two dogs with hip dysplasia and osteoarthritis (Fig. 2). One disease-free dog served as a control. Compared to the surrounding cartilage on the femoral head surface, collagen deposition into cartilage was decreased (40%) in the focal region where the cartilage surface was fibrillated (Figs 1 and 2). In the control joints obtained from the disease-free dog the synthesis of collagen at the site of lesion predilection was similar to that in its surrounding cartilage.

One dysplastic dog that was injected intravenously with ^{3}H-proline not only had hip osteoarthritis, but at necropsy also had fibrillated cartilage on both medial tibial plateaus. Collagen deposition was diminished in the fibrillated regions in both knee joints. The shoulders of this dog were disease free and the sites of lesion predilection on the humeral heads did not have a

60

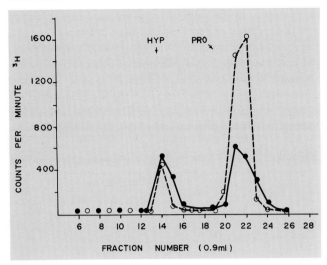

Fig. 2. Incorporation *in vivo* of ³H-proline into collagen and non-collagenous protein in the articular cartilage of a femoral head of a hip joint from a dog with hip dysplasia and cartilage degeneration. ³H-proline injected intravenously for 60 hours prior to necropsy. Degenerated and 'unaffected' surrounding cartilage was collected. Degenerated and normal cartilage (9 mg of each, dry weight) were hydrolysed in 6 M HCl and ³H-proline and ³H-hydroxyproline separated by ion exchange chromatography. ●——● data from 'normal' surrounding cartilage; ○– – –○ degenerated cartilage. Data as counts per minute.

decreased rate of collagen deposition when compared to the surrounding humeral head cartilage.

Loss of proteoglycans and collagen from articular cartilage is a feature of the osteoarthritic process. A study of electron micrographs showed that degenerated cartilage taken from the joints of dogs with hip dysplasia had collagen fibres that were disoriented (e.g. loss of characteristic banding pattern) and of smaller diameter (Wiltberger and Lust, 1975). In fact, very early signs of injury to the cartilage include focal defects in the layer covering the cartilage surface and the loosening and exposure of the collagen fibrils and bundles (Greisen *et al.*, 1982).

Ehrlich *et al.* (1978) reported increased collagenase levels in osteoarthritic cartilage from humans, and Pelletier *et al.* (1983) confirmed these results. Increased collagenolytic activity also was observed in canine fibrillated cartilage (Wurster *et al.*, 1982). Taken together these data are suggestive of increased collagenase activity in the matrix, but other possibilities exist. Berg *et al.* (1981) reported that from 20 to 40% of newly synthesised collagen can be destroyed intracellularly within minutes of being synthesised, possibly the result of a normal process by which the cell can modulate the quantity and quality of the collagen being secreted from it. That this process is for some reason altered in the degenerated cartilage must also be considered.

In this disease the 'normal' cartilage surrounding the site of fibrillation resembles normal cartilage taken from a disease-free joint. This was not true of the surgically induced osteoarthritis of the knee studied by Eyre *et al.* (1980) and Floman *et al.* (1980). They suggested that an increase in synthesis was observed in all the cartilage from the affected joint.

These disparities are unexplained, though several possibilities have been suggested by ourselves and others. First, our studies in dogs have focused on very early changes that occur in the cartilage, often in advance of clinical disease and before changes in the joint can be detected by radiological methods. At this time, focal areas of cartilage degeneration can be discerned.

Our studies of collagen content, deposition, and synthesis have, for the most part, involved comparisons of the fibrillated cartilage and morphologically normal tissue obtained from outlying regions of the same cartilage. The conflicting data reported by others have often been based on measurements of collagen metabolism in the whole cartilage, comparisons being made with tissue obtained from apparently unaffected joints. Differences may be related to sampling within and between joints. To this may be added variation between subjects, differences in animal species, and variations in collagen metabolism that may occur at different stages of the disease process. It remains to be seen whether these variables can explain the inconsistencies.

We have used both *in vivo* and *in vitro* labelling methods to document diminished collagen deposition in lesions as measured by the conversion of proline to hydroxyproline. We are confident that our data are sound and that the conclusions drawn are valid for the dog and the early stage of the disease. We are encouraged further by similar studies showing diminished collagen deposition in the degenerated cartilage obtained from joints other than the hip. All of these studies pertaining to collagen metabolism suggest that, although collagen deposition is reduced at the site of fibrillation, the surrounding cartilage is metabolically similar to cartilage obtained from a normal joint. This would be consistent with our study of the glycosaminoglycan content of cartilage, in which we found that it too was similar in disease-free joints and in 'normal' areas of cartilage from young dogs whose joints exhibit early osteoarthritic changes (Lust and Pronsky, 1972).

Although the observed changes in collagen begin in focal areas, the process extends to involve the entire cartilage. Our own data, and those of others, suggest that a derangement of collagen metabolism or collagen structure is linked in some way to fibrillation of the articular cartilage. Whether the observed changes are causally related to osteoarthritis or are a response to another, as yet unidentified, mechanism is unknown. Nevertheless, further studies of events which precede, accompany and follow the observed changes in cartilage collagen metabolism are expected to cast new light on the disease process.

Fibronectin of articular cartilage

Fibronectin is a protein of extracellular matrices and this interesting molecule functions in cell adhesion, migration, morphology, differentiation, metabolism and transformation (Rouslahti *et al.*, 1981). Fibronectin was present in low amounts in disease-free dog cartilage (Table II). The quantities extracted from normal cartilage (using canine plasma fibronectin in an ELISA test (Wurster and Lust, 1982) were about 80 ng/mg wet cartilage. A striking finding was that substantially greater amounts of fibronectin were extracted from degenerated (i.e. fibrillated) cartilage: as much as 3600 ng/mg tissue from the severely degenerated cartilage of a seven-year-old arthritic dog (Table II).

Table II. Fibronectin content in normal and osteoarthritic articular cartilage

Source of cartilage	Fibronectin content[a] (ng/mg wet cartilage)
Disease-free joint (6-month dog)	80
Osteoarthritic joint (6-month dog)	
Surrounding region	90
Focal degeneration	1000
Degenerated (7-year dog)	3600

[a]Fibronectin was extracted with a buffer that contained heparin and urea (Wurster and Lust, 1982). The use of harsher procedures for disruption, including 4 M guanidinium chloride and collagenase treatment, extracted additional quantities of fibronectin from the articular cartilage.

From the interpretations of Dessau et al. (1978) it may be that fibronectin accumulated as a consequence of the loss of matrix material (e.g. protoeoglycans) which accompanies the osteoarthritic process. The accumulated fibronectin may have no further role in the osteoarthritic process. However, since fibronectin affects the morphology and the differentiation of chondrocytes and reduces proteoglycan synthesis (Pennypacker et al., 1979), it is plausible to think that the local presence of fibronectin favours the progression of the disease, possibly impeding repair of damaged cartilage in some way.

Methods of tissue disruption, including extraction with 5 M guanidinium chloride and collagenase treatment, have substantiated the findings shown in Table II, that degenerated cartilages from osteoarthritic canine joints contain more fibronectin (Wurster and Lust, 1983). Furthermore, incubation of cartilage explants in vitro with ^{3}H-phenylalanine and determination of radioactivity in the fibronectin isolated on gelatin affinity columns or by SDS-PAGE revealed that both normal and degenerated cartilage explants were able to synthesise fibronectin. Some of the newly made fibronectin was transferred into the incubation medium (Wurster and Lust, 1983). Fibronectin in cartilage in vivo could originate from the chondrocytes or alternatively from the synoviocytes of the synovium via the synovial fluid. Experiments to date cannot resolve this question, but they reveal that chondrocytes of cartilage explants in vitro possess the ability to synthesise fibronectin.

The fibronectin concentrations of dog plasma and synovial

fluids are presented in Table III. The plasma content of osteoarthritic dogs was not changed compared to disease-free dogs; but the synovial fluid concentration was elevated substantially in osteoarthritic joints. Further studies must delineate whether the increased concentration of fibronectin in the fluid from osteoarthritic joints is the source of the elevated content of fibronectin in fibrillated cartilage, or whether the cartilage and synovial fluid fibronectins are indeed different molecules.

Table III. Fibronectin concentration of dog plasma and synovial fluid

	Fibronectin μg/ml (means $\pm$ s.d.)
Plasma[a]	
Disease-free dogs (5)	955 ± 211
Osteoarthritic dogs (7)	927 ± 262
Synovial fluid[b]	
Disease-free joints (9)	91 ± 15
Osteoarthritic joints (9)	480 ± 410

[a]Based on radiographic examination of hip joint; human plasma contains 300–400 μg/ml fibronectin.
[b]Based on necropsy examination of joints, i.e. volume of fluid and condition of articular cartilage.

It has been reported that fibronectin is not present in the matrix of a mature cartilage (Rouslahti et al., 1981; Dessau et al., 1978) although chondrocytes synthesised fibronectin when the matrix environment was altered (Dessau et al., 1978). The presence of proteoglycan in the extracellular matrix may make the detection of fibronectin in cartilage difficult (Weiss and Reddi, 1981) and be responsible for reports of its absence.

Unidentified, non-collagenous proteins have been described in several reports. Labelling the cartilage of an osteoarthritic joint by intravenous injection of ^{3}H-proline resulted in a five-fold increase in the accumulation of ^{3}H-proline into a non-collagenous substance in the fibrillated area as opposed to the surrounding, unaffected cartilage (Fig. 2). This ^{3}H-proline was shown to be precipitable by 67% ethanol and sensitive to trypsin, suggesting it was in protein (Wurster et al., 1982). Increased synthesis of non-collagenous protein in osteoarthritic cartilage from human patients was reported by Miller and Mankin (1982), and in dogs with experimentally induced osteoarthritis by Eyre et al. (1980). Also, when cultured under conditions in which collagenous synthesis was selectively inhibited, fibroblasts showed increased synthesis of a non-collagenous protein (Jiminez et al., 1979). Electron micrographs of fibrillated cartilage taken from joints of dogs with hip dysplasia disclosed the accumulation of a densely-staining amorphous material dispersed among the collagen fibres in the matrix (Lust et al., 1972; Wiltberger and Lust, 1975). These materials have not yet been characterised but the possibility that they are fibronectin or products derived from it must be considered.

ACKNOWLEDGEMENTS

The authors' research was supported in part by the late John M. Olin, the Kroc Foundation, and NIH Grant AM 20665. The collaboration of H.A. Greisen, S.J. Harter, J.M. Olsewski, V.T. Rendano, A. Signore and B.A. Summers is gratefully acknowledged.

REFERENCES

ADAMS, M.E. and BILLINGHAM, M.E.J. (1982) Animal models of osteoarthritis. In: *Current Topics in Pathology*, Vol. 71, C.L. Berry (Ed.), pp. 265–297. Springer, Berlin.

BERG, R.A., SCHWARTZ, M.L. and CRYSTAL, R.G. (1981) Regulation of the production of secretory proteins; intracellular degradation of newly synthesised defective collagen. *Proc. Natl. Acad. Sci. USA* **77**, 4746–4756.

BYERS, P.D., MAROUDAS, A., OZTOP, F., STOCKWELL, R.A. and VENN, M. (1977) Histological and biochemical studies on cartilage from osteoarthrotic femoral heads with special reference to surface characteristics. *Connect. Tissue Res.* **5**, 41–49.

COOKE, T.D.V., BENNETT, E.L. and OHRO, O. (1980) Identification of immunoglobulins and complement components in articular cartilage of patients with idiopathic osteoarthritis. In: *Aetiopathogenesis of Osteoarthrosis*, G. Nuki (Ed.), pp. 144–154. Pitman Medical, Tunbridge Wells.

DESSAU, W., SASSE, J., TIMPL, R., JILEK, F. and VON DER MARK, F. (1978) Synthesis and extracellular deposition of fibronectin in chondrocyte cultures. Response to the removal of extracellular cartilage matrix. *J. Cell Biol.* **79**, 342–355.

EHRLICH, M.G., HOULE, P.A., VIGLIANI, G. and MANKIN, H.J. (1978) Correlation between articular cartilage collagenase activity and osteoarthritis. *Arthritis Rheum.* **21**, 761–766.

EYRE, D.R., McDEVITT, C.A., BILLINGHAM, E.J. and MUIR, H. (1980) Biosynthesis of collagen and other matrix proteins by articular cartilage in experimental osteoarthrosis. *Biochem. J.* **188**, 823–837.

FLOMAN, Y., EYRE, D.R. and GLIMCHER, M.J. (1980) Induction of osteoarthrosis in the rabbit knee joint: biochemical studies on the articular cartilage. *Clin. Orthop. Rel. Res.* **147**, 278–286.

GREISEN, H.A., SUMMERS, B.A. and LUST, G. (1982) Ultrastructure of the articular cartilage and synovium in the early stages of degenerative joint disease in canine hip joints. *Am. J. Vet. Res.* **43**, 1963–1971.

HEWITT, A.T., KLEINMAN, H.K., PENNYPACKER, J.P. and MARTIN, G.R. (1980) Identification of an adhesion factor for chondrocytes. *Proc. Natl. Acad. Sci. USA* **77**, 385–388.

HUI-CHOU, C. and LUST, G. (1982) The type of collagen made by the articular cartilage in joints of dogs with osteoarthritis. *Coll. Rel. Res.* **2**, 245–256.

HUSKISSON, E.C., DIEPPE, P.A., TUCKER, A.K. and CANNELL, L.B. (1979) Another look at osteoarthritis. *Ann. Rheum. Dis.* **38**, 423–428.

JIMINEZ, S.A., McARTHUR, W. and ROSENBLOOM, J. (1979) Inhibition of collagen synthesis by mononuclear cell supernates. *J. Exp. Med.* **50**, 142–153.

KELLGREN, J.H. and MOORE, G. (1952) Generalised osteoarthritis and Heberden's nodes. *Br. Med. J.* **1**, 181–187.

LUST, G., BEILMAN, W.T. and RENDANO, V.T. (1980) A relationship between degree of laxity and synovial fluid volume in coxofemoral joints of dogs predisposed for hip dysplasia. *Am. J. Vet. Res.* **41**, 55–60.

LUST, G. and PRONSKY, W. (1972) Glycosaminoglycan contents of normal and degenerative articular cartilage from dogs. *Clin. Chim. Acta* **39**, 281–286.

LUST, G., PRONSKY, W. and SHERMAN, D.M. (1972) Biochemical and ultrastructural observations in normal and degenerative canine articular cartilage. *Am. J. Vet. Res.* **33**, 2429–2445.

LUST, G. and SUMMERS, B.A. (1981) Early, asymptomatic stage of degenerative joint disease in canine hip joints. *Am. J. Vet. Res.* **42**, 1849–1855.

MANKIN, H.J., JOHNSON, M.E. and LIPPIELLO, L. (1981) Biochemical and metabolic abnormalities in articular cartilage from osteoarthritic human hips. III. Distribution and metabolism of amino sugar-containing molecules. *J. Bone Joint Surg.* **63**A, 131–139.

MILLER, D.R. and MANKIN, H.J. (1982) Abstract. *Trans. Orthop. Res. Soc.* **7**, 91.

MOSKOWITZ, R.W., GOLDBERG, V.M. and MALEMUD, C.J. (1981) Metabolic responses of cartilage in experimentally induced osteoarthritis. *Ann. Rheum. Dis.* **40**, 584–592.

NIMNI, M.E. and DESHMUKH, K. (1973) Differences in collagen metabolism between normal and osteoarthritic human articular cartilage. *Science* **181**, 751–752.

OLSEWSKI, J.M., LUST, G., RENDANO, V.T. and SUMMERS, B.A. (1983) Degenerative joint disease: Multiple joint involvement in young and mature dogs. *Am. J. Vet. Res.* **44**, 1300–1308.

PAULSSON, M. and HEINEGÅRD, D. (1981) Purification and structural characterisation of a cartilage matrix protein. *Biochem. J.* **197**, 367–375.

PEDERSON, N.C. and POOL, R. (1978) Canine degenerative joint disease. *Vet. Clin. North Am.* **8**, 465–493.

PELLETIER, J.-P., MARTEL-PELLETIER, J., HOWELL, D.S., GHANDUR-MNAYMNEH, L., ENIS, J.E. and WOESSNER, J.F. Jr (1983) Collagenase and collagenolytic activity in human osteoarthritic cartilage. *Arthritis Rheum.* **26**, 63–68.

PENNYPACKER, J.P., HASSELL, J.R., YAMADA, K.M. and PRATT, R.M. (1979) The influence of an adhesive cell surface protein on chondrogenic expression *in vitro. Exp. Cell Res.* **121**, 411–415.

ROUSLAHTI, E., ENGVALL, E. and HAYMAN, E.G. (1981) Fibronectin: Current concepts of its structure and function. *Coll. Rel. Res.* **1**, 95–128.

WEISS, R.E. and REDDI, A.H. (1981) Role of fibronectin in collagenous matrix-induced mesenchymal cell proliferation and differentiation *in vivo*. *Exp. Cell Res.* **133**(2), 247–254.

WILTBERGER, H. and LUST, G. (1975) Ultrastructure of canine articular cartilage: comparison of normal and degenerative (osteoarthritic) hip joints. *Am. J. Vet. Res.* **36**, 727–740.

WURSTER, N.B., HUI-CHOU, C.S., GREISEN, H.A. and LUST, G. (1982) Reduced deposition of collagen in the degenerated articular cartilage of dogs with degenerative joint disease. *Biochim. Biophys. Acta* **718**, 74–84.

WURSTER, N.B. and LUST, G. (1982) Fibronectin in osteoarthritic canine articular cartilage. *Biochim. Biophys. Res. Commun.* **109**, 1094–1101.

WURSTER, N.B. and LUST, G. (1983) Fibronectin content and biosynthesis in normal and osteoarthritic canine articular cartilage. *Fed. Proc.* **42**, 1843 (Abstract).

YAZICI, H., SAVILLE, P.D., SALVATI, E., BOHARE, W. and WILSON, P. (1975) Primary osteoarthrosis of the knee or hip. Prevalence of Heberden nodes in relation to age and sex. *JAMA* **231**, 1256–1260.

64

Chapter 5

Cellular Changes in Synovium and Meniscus of a Rabbit Model of Osteoarthritis induced by Partial Meniscectomy

D. C. SWARTZENDRUBER, C. COLOMBO, M. BUTLER, L. HICKMAN, M. WOODWORTH and B. G. STEINETZ

Research Department, Pharmaceuticals Division, CIBA-GEIGY Corporation, Ardsley, New York, USA

SUMMARY

Partial meniscectomy in the rabbit knee joint leads within six weeks to changes resembling those of osteoarthritis in man. The pathological features are reproducible, and severity of lesion can be assessed by scoring histological and histochemical changes and by measuring uptake of the radionuclide gallium-67 (^{67}Ga). The contralateral joint is sham-operated or non-operated and serves as control.

Histological assessment is based on degree of structural change, staining characteristics, loss or disorganisation of chondrocytes, cluster formation, loss of cartilage, osteophyte development, and bony change. ^{67}Ga is localised in lysosomes to an extent correlating with enzyme activity: in this rabbit model ^{67}Ga uptake is increased after partial meniscectomy, suggesting raised enzyme levels and their possible role in cartilage degeneration. Studies of the protease cathepsin B, which degrades proteoglycan, showed raised concentrations in hyperplastic synovium from operated knees. The synovium becomes hyperplastic and inflamed within three weeks of surgery but these changes are less marked at six weeks: synovial cells may therefore be actively involved in the production of factors inducing early cartilage destruction.

This model is being employed to study potentially useful drugs for treatment of osteoarthritis in man.

INTRODUCTION

A partial lateral meniscectomy procedure has been used to induce a condition resembling osteoarthritis (OA) in the knees of rabbits (Colombo *et al.*, 1983b). This involves section of the fibular collateral and sesamoid ligaments and removal of 4–5 mm of the anterior lateral meniscus. Significant pathology develops in the tibial and femoral articular cartilage six weeks after surgery. Cartilage and bone lesions from surgical controls and drug-treated rabbits are evaluated histologically and the scores compared as a measure of efficacy. This model is used to detect potentially useful drugs for treatment of human OA (Colombo *et al.*, 1983b; Steinetz *et al.*, 1983).

The induced disease is due in part to mechanical factors caused by joint instability. Cellular and biochemical factors such as synthesis and release of cartilage-degrading substances (proteoglycanases, collagenases and other mediators which stimulate chondrocytes to release active proteases) by traumatised tissue, i.e. meniscus and synovium, may also contribute to the development of articular cartilage lesions in this model. Recent studies have focused on cellular changes in the meniscus and synovium by measuring uptake of the radionuclide ^{67}Ga and by histochemical localisation of cathepsin B.

SURGICAL PROCEDURE

Adult male New Zealand rabbits weighing approximately four kilograms were subjected to a partial lateral meniscectomy procedure as described by Colombo *et al.* (1983b). Briefly, the procedure involved section of the fibular collateral and sesamoid ligaments and removal of 4–5 mm of the anterior lateral meniscus. The surgical procedure is a modification of the Moskowitz *et al.* (1973) and Telhag and Lindberg (1972) methods of inducing experimental OA. The operation was performed on the right knee, the contralateral knee serving as a control. Sham operations consisted of cutting through the skin and exposing the ligaments and meniscus.

GALLIUM-67-CITRATE UPTAKE

The radiopharmaceutical, gallium-67 citrate (^{67}Ga citrate), was obtained from New England Nuclear. A dose of 300–400 μCi was injected intraperitoneally 24 hours before the animals were killed. A total of 40 rabbits were killed at one, three, six and 12 weeks after surgery. Four non-operated rabbits and four sham-operated rabbits were also used in these experiments. Selected tissues were removed, weighed and assayed for radioactivity in a Beckman Gamma 8000 counting system. Tissue ratios of ^{67}Ga uptake were calculated for operated as against contralateral knees. Tissues were assayed in scintillation vials containing fixative which allowed them to be processed later for histopathological study.

PROCESSING OF TISSUES FOR MORPHOLOGICAL STUDIES

Samples of tibial and femoral cartilage attached to the underlying subchondral bone, the patella, the remaining lateral meniscus, the medial meniscus, and the infrapatellar fat pad with attached synovial membrane were removed for the time-course study. For drug-testing purposes, only femoral and articular cartilage samples were removed and processed, as described earlier (Colombo *et al.*, 1983b). For routine histological study, tissues were immersed immediately in 10% formalin containing 1% sodium acetate and 7% EDTA (pH 5·2) and allowed to decalcify in paraffin wax. Tissue sections were cut at 6 μm and stained with safranin 0 and fast green.

Samples of tissues for electron microscopy were fixed in a modified Karnovsky (1965) fixative, post-fixed in 2% osmium tetroxide buffered with sodium cacodylate and embedded in Polybed 812. Thin sections were stained with a 50:50 mixture of aqueous uranyl acetate and acetone, washed, and stained with lead citrate.

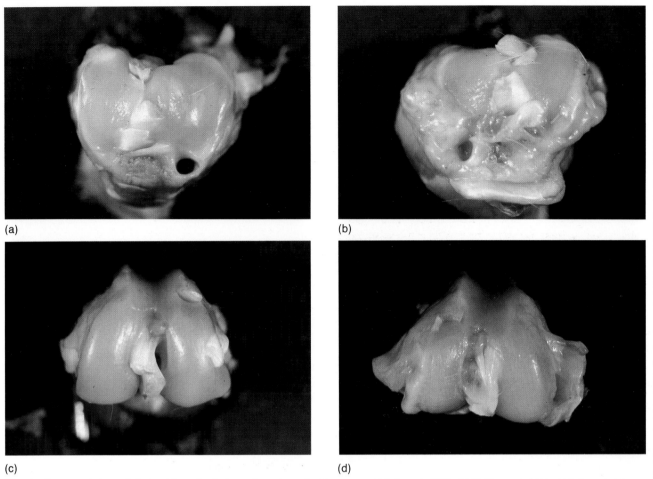

(a)

(b)

(c)

(d)

Fig. 1. Gross morphology of tibial and femoral articular cartilage six weeks after surgery. (a) Left, control tibia. (b) Right, operated tibia. (c) Left, control femur. (d) Right, operated femur.

HISTOCHEMICAL STUDIES

Synovial and meniscal samples for histochemical studies were embedded in Tissue Tek II OCT Embedding Compound (Miles Laboratories) and frozen immediately in liquid-nitrogen-chilled isopentane and stored at −70°C. Sections 10 μm thick were cut in a cryostat, picked up on acid-cleaned cover slips and fixed in 2% cacodylate-buffered glutaraldehyde, following the enzyme histochemical fluorescence technique described by Graf *et al.* (1981) to localise cathepsin B. The method is based on the reaction principle that cathepsin B cleaves the substrate N-CBZ-L-Ala-L-Arg-L-Arg-2-(4-methoxy)naphthylamide 2HCl(Z-Ala-Arg-Arg-MNA) and also liberates 2-(4-methoxy)naphthylamine (MNA), which is trapped by 5-nitrosalicylaldehyde (NSA) as a fine particulate fluorescent complex. Fixed sections were incubated in the substrate for 10–30 minutes, nuclei were counterstained with ethidium bromide, and the sections mounted and photographed within three hours. Sections of mouse heart were used to monitor the reaction, and other sections which were incubated without substrate or in the presence of leupeptin, an

inhibitor of cathepsin B, were examined as controls.

For fluorescence microscopy, a Zeiss photomicroscope equipped with vertical illuminator III RS and HBO 50 mercury lamp was used. The filter combinations were UVG 365, a broad-band exciter filter at 300–400 nm, reflector at 395 nm, and barrier filter at 420 nm.

RESULTS

The rabbit model of OA was designed primarily as a secondary screen in a drug development programme. Gross lesions are observed (Fig. 1) and recorded but the use of the model in the screening programme relies heavily on histological evaluation of articular cartilage sections six weeks after surgery. Consistent, reproducible lesions (Fig. 2) occur at this end-point and are scored on a 0–4 grading scale. Total lesion scores are determined for each group of animals within an experiment. Details of the

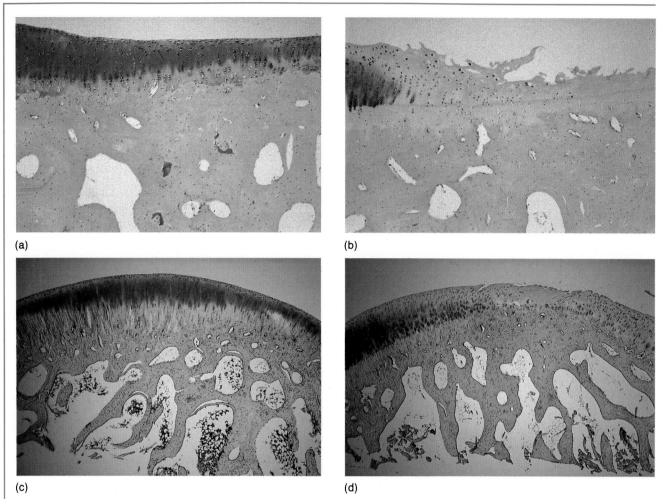

Fig. 2. Histological appearance of articular cartilage six weeks after surgery. (a) Left, control tibia. (b) Right, operated tibia. Note lack of safranin uptake, fibrillation, disorganisation and loss of chondrocytes, and loss of cartilage. (c) Left, control femur. (d) Right, operated femur. Note typical pathological lesions. (Safranin 0 and fast green.)

drug-screening programme have been presented elsewhere (Colombo *et al.*, 1983a; Steinetz *et al.*, 1987). See Chapter 7.

The histological evaluation of the model is admittedly subjective, and we are continually seeking methods to improve the scoring system. These include revising the number of lesions scored, to avoid weighting of certain lesions, and combining and/or deleting lesions that have high correlations in their occurrence or that occur very infrequently. In order to facilitate this procedure we have computerised the model. As a result of the initial analysis we have proposed a new system that incorporates eight lesions. These are reduced from the original 12 used in the development of the model. The new system (Table I), assigns higher values to progressive stages of lesion development, e.g. alterations in the superficial cartilage layer that precede 'fibrillation' receive a score of 1, whereas putative progressive changes receive higher scores. Shapiro and Glimcher (1980) made similar attempts to quantitate lesion severity in an experimental OA model, modifying Mankin's (1973) classification system.

Another approach that might be applicable for quantitation of lesion scores is the use of radionuclide joint imaging (Hoffer and Genant, 1976). Surprisingly few dynamic radiotracer studies have been done on experimental arthritis models (Bohr, 1976), considering the wide applications of these modern techniques in clinical rheumatology.

We evaluated the uptake of ^{67}Ga citrate in rabbit knee-joint tissues at one, three, six, and 12 weeks after surgery. Significant differences in ^{67}Ga ratios were observed in synovium and meniscus at the one- and three-week intervals (Figs 3 and 4). The right (operated) synovium showed an eight-fold increase at one week; this decreased to approximately six-fold at three weeks and returned to control values at six and 12 weeks after surgery. The right meniscus showed a similar pattern of ^{67}Ga uptake.

The exact mechanism of ^{67}Ga-citrate localisation is unknown, but it takes place in lysosomes (Swartzendruber *et al.*, 1971), and its localisation in lysosomes has been correlated with the

68

Table I. System used for scoring histological changes in cartilage

Lesion	Score				
	0	1	2	3	4
Structural changes	None	Loss of superficial layer	Moderate fibrillation	Extensive fibrillation	Cartilage erosion
Loss of safranin O staining	None	Paler than control	Moderate loss	Marked loss	Total loss
Loss of chondrocytes	None	Slight decrease	Moderate decrease	Marked decrease	Extensive hypocellularity
Loss of cartilage	None	Slight loss	Moderate loss	Marked loss	Loss of cartilage to bone
Chondrocyte clusters ('clones')	None	Few 3–4 small or 1–2 medium	Several 5–6 small or 3–4 medium or 1–2 large	Many 7–8 small or 5–6 medium or 3–4 large	Very many 9+ small or 7–8 medium or 5–6 large
Osteophytes	None	Very small	Small	Medium	Large
Disorganisation of chondrocytes	None	Noticeable	Moderate Some loss of columns	Marked loss of columns	No recogniseable organisation
Bone changes	None	Slight increase in capillaries	Moderate increase in capillaries	Marked increase in capillaries	Capillaries penetrate the tide mark

activities of four hydrolytic enzymes: aryl sulphatase, beta-glucuronidase, acid phosphatase and cathepsin D (Hammersley and Taylor, 1979). The high uptake of ^{67}Ga citrate in the traumatised synovium and meniscus of the rabbit model suggests that increased levels of hydrolytic enzymes are present in these tissues. These cellular products may play a role in cartilage degeneration in this model, as was shown by *in vitro* synovium-cartilage studies by Fell and Jubb (1977).

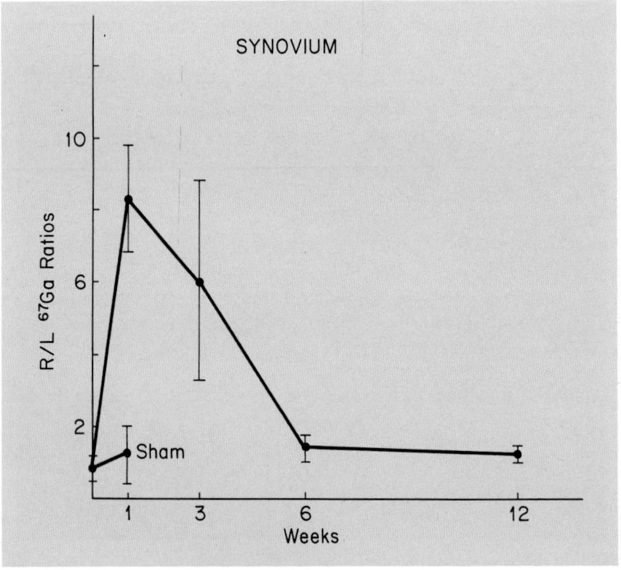

Histological study of the synovial membrane of the operated knee at one and three weeks after surgery in the rabbit model shows synovial-cell hyperplasia, infiltration by polymorphonuclear leucocytes, increased numbers of congested blood

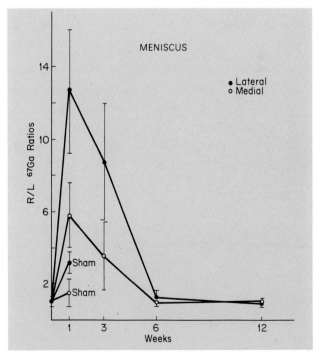

Fig. 3. Ratio of ^{67}Ga uptake in synovia of operated versus contralateral knee joints as a function of time after surgery.

Fig. 4. Ratio of ^{67}Ga uptake in menisci of operated versus contralateral knee joints as a function of time after surgery. Note increase in ^{67}Ga uptake in the medial meniscus in addition to the surgically-operated lateral meniscus.

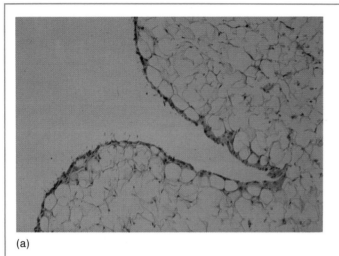

(a)

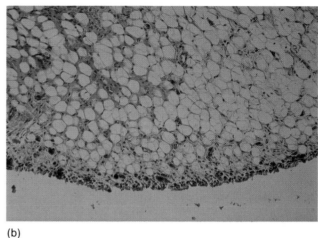

(b)

Fig. 5. Histological appearance of synovial membrane. (a) Control (left knee). (b) Right knee three weeks after surgery. Note the synovial-cell hyperplasia, fibrosis, increased vascularisation and polymorphonuclear infiltration. (Haematoxylin and eosin.)

vessels and varying amounts of fibrosis (Fig. 5). Many cells in the hyperplastic synovial membrane contain an elaborate rough-surfaced endoplasmic reticulum, numerous small electron-dense bodies (possibly lysosomes) and a prominent Golgi complex (Fig. 6). These cytoplasmic features are characteristic of actively synthesising and secreting cells.

Similar cells were observed on the surface of the remaining right lateral meniscus (Fig. 7) at three and six weeks after surgery. These cells were accompanied by numerous blood vessels and appeared to be an extension of the synovial membrane.

Cathepsin B, a thiol-dependent protease that can degrade proteoglycan at near-neutral pH, was localised in cells in the synovial membrane (Fig. 8). Cathepsin B activity was present

Fig. 6. Electron micrograph of a synoviocyte from the right knee of a rabbit three weeks after surgery. Note the rough-surfaced endoplasmic reticulum and the small membrane-bound dense (lysosome-like) bodies in the cytoplasm. Profiles of the smooth membranes of the Golgi apparatus are present near the indented nucleus.

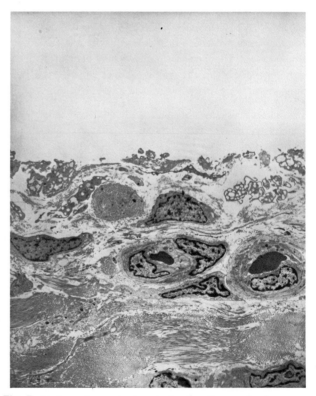

Fig. 7. Electron micrograph of meniscal surface three weeks after surgery, showing blood vessels and cells with extensive rough-surfaced endoplasmic reticulum similar to synoviocytes. Note bundles of collagen below the blood vessels.

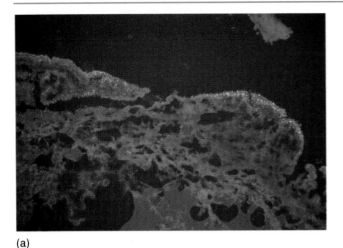
(a)

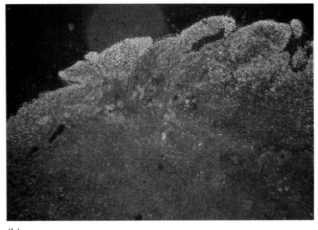
(b)

Fig. 8. Fluorescence localisation of cathepsin B in synovium six weeks after surgery. (a) Left, control knee. (b) Right, operated knee, six weeks after surgery. Note increased amount in the right synovium.

in synovium from contralateral unoperated knees but was increased in the hyperplastic synovium of the operated knees and also in the overlying cells on the meniscal surface at three and six weeks after surgery (Fig. 9).

The synovial membrane in the rabbit model was less hyperplastic, with varying amounts of fibrosis six weeks after surgery. The transient inflammatory phase shown histologically and by increased ^{67}Ga-citrate uptake occurs early in the course of the disease (1–3 weeks after surgery). It is not clear whether the transient synovitis induces or stimulates degenerative changes in cartilage or is a secondary change. Muckle (1982) suggested that knee-joint instability of OA animal models produced degenerative cartilage lesions that stimulated secondary synovial changes, but this is not clearly established.

Classically, osteoarthritis is considered to be a non-inflammatory disease although there is low-level inflammation in many cases. Only a few studies have been reported on synovial changes in the early intervals after surgery in experimental models. Studies of animal models of OA induced by partial meniscectomy procedures have generally focused on cartilage degeneration at 2–3 months after surgery. Champion and Poole (1982) stated that a period of acute inflammation occurred in joints of rabbits that had undergone meniscectomy. McDevitt *et al.* (1977) also reported inflammatory changes in experimentally induced OA in dogs.

We have shown a high uptake of ^{67}Ga citrate in the synovium and meniscus at one and three weeks after surgery, synovial-cell hyperplasia with morphological changes characteristic of actively synthesising cells, and increased levels of cathepsin B in the synovium at these early times following surgery.

These results suggest that synovial cells are actively involved in the production of factors that may bring about the degradation of cartilage in the surgically-induced rabbit model of OA. The evaluation of drug effects on these early cellular changes

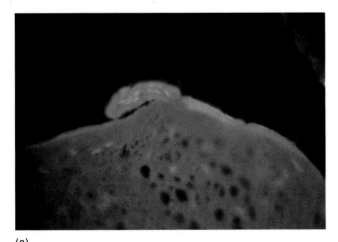
(a)

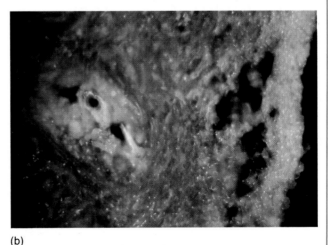
(b)

Fig. 9. Fluorescence localisation of cathepsin B six weeks after surgery in: (a) Left, control meniscus, and (b) Right, operated meniscus. Note lack of activity in left meniscus and intense activity in the overgrowing cells on the meniscal surface.

71

in the synovium may provide another end-point in the search for potentially effective drugs.

REFERENCES

BOHR, N. (1976) Experimental osteoarthritis in the rabbit knee joint. *Acta Orthop. Scand.* **47**, 558–565.

CHAMPION, B.R. and POOLE, A.R. (1982) Immunity to homologous type III collagen after partial meniscectomy and sham surgery in rabbits. *Arthritis Rheum.* **25**, 274–287.

COLOMBO, C., BUTLER, M., HICKMAN, L., SELWYN, M., CHART, J. and STEINETZ, B. (1983a) A new model of osteoarthritis in rabbits. II. Evaluation of anti-osteoarthritic effects of selected antirheumatic drugs administered systemically. *Arthritis Rheum.* **26**, 1132–1139.

COLOMBO, C., BUTLER, M., O'BYRNE, E., HICKMAN, L., SWARTZENDRUBER, D., SELWYN, M. and STEINETZ, B. (1983b) A new model of osteoarthritis in rabbits. I. Development of knee joint pathology following lateral meniscectomy and section of the fibular collateral and sesamoid ligaments. *Arthritis Rheum.* **26**, 875–886.

FELL, H.B. and JUBB, R.W. (1977) The effect of synovial tissue on the breakdown of articular cartilage in organ culture. *Arthritis Rheum.* **20**, 1359–1371.

GRAF, M., BAICI, A. and STRÄULI, P. (1981) Histochemical localisation of cathepsin B at the invasion front of the rabbit v2 carcinoma. *Lab. Invest.* **45**, 587–596.

HAMMERSLEY, P.A.G. and TAYLOR, D.M. (1979) The role of lysosomal enzyme activity in the localisation of ^{67}Ga-citrate. *Eur. J. Nucl. Med.* **4**, 261–270.

HOFFER, P.B. and GENANT, N.K. (1976) Radionuclide joint imaging. *Semin. Nucl. Med.* **6**, 121–137.

KARNOVSKY, M.J. (1965) A formaldehyde–glutaraldehyde fixative of high osmolarity for use in electron microscopy. *J. Cell Biol.* **27**, 137A.

MANKIN, H.J. (1973) Biochemical and metabolic abnormalities in osteoarthritic human cartilage. *Fed. Proc.* **32**, 1478–1480.

McDEVITT, C., GILBERTSON, E. and MUIR, H. (1977) An experimental model of osteoarthritis; early morphological and biochemical changes. *J. Bone Joint Surg.* **59**B, 24–35.

MOSKOWITZ, R.W., DAVIS, W., SAMMARCO, J., MARTENS, M., BAKER, J., MAYER, M., BURSTEIN, A.H. and FRANKEL, V.N. (1973) Experimentally induced degenerative joint lesions following partial meniscectomy in the rabbit. *Arthritis Rheum.* **16**, 397–405.

MUCKLE, D.S. (1982) Inflammatory involvement in osteoarthritis and lessons to be learnt from animal models. *Eur. J. Rheum. Inflamm.* **5**, 39–45.

SHAPIRO, F. and GLIMCHER, M.J. (1980) Induction of osteoarthrosis in the rabbit knee joint: Histologic changes following meniscectomy and meniscal lesions. *Clin. Orthop.* **147**, 287–295.

STEINETZ, B.G., COLOMBO, C., BUTLER, M., O'BYRNE, E.M. and STEELE, R.E. (1981) Animal models of osteoarthritis: Possible application in a drug development program. *Curr. Ther. Res.* **30**, S60–S75.

STEINETZ, B.G., COLOMBO, C., BUTLER, M., O'BYRNE, E.M., HICKMAN, L.Y. and SWARTZENDRUBER, D.C. (1987) Effect of selected antirheumatic agents on surgically induced degenerative knee joint disease in rabbit. This volume.

SWARTZENDRUBER, D.C., NELSON, B. and HAYES, R.L. (1971) Gallium-67 localisation in lysosomal-like granules of leukemic and nonleukemic murine tissues. *J. Nat. Cancer Inst.* **46**, 941–952.

TELHAG, N. and LINDBERG, L. (1972) A method for inducing osteoarthritic changes in rabbits' knees. *Clin. Orthop.* **86**, 214–223.

EFFECTS OF INTERVENTION ON THE PROCESSES OF OA

Chapter 6

Osteoarthrosis-like Disease in Mice: Effects of Anti-arthrotic and Anti-rheumatic Agents

RENÉ MAIER and GERHARD WILHELMI

Research Department, Pharmaceuticals Division, CIBA-GEIGY Ltd, Basle, Switzerland

SUMMARY

The effects of a number of non-steroidal anti-inflammatory drugs have been studied in the spontaneous osteoarthritis which arises in the C57 black mouse. In this model, characteristic joint changes take place progressively from about six months of age, providing a firm basis for assessing the effects of intervention.

In the first study reported below, the affected joints were counted and severity of lesions graded on an arbitrary scale (+ to + + + +), mostly after four months' treatment with several different agents. The incidence of arthrotic joints tended to be less frequent with all the 'anti-arthrotic' drugs tested (except glucosamine sulphate in low dosage), and the severity of the lesions less pronounced with all but polysulphated glycosaminoglycans and glucosamine sulphate.

Of the anti-inflammatory drugs given to relieve pain during acute episodes, prednisone accelerated the spontaneous degeneration, as expected, but so also did naproxen, ibuprofen, acetylsalicylic acid and phenylbutazone. Indomethacin on the whole and pirprofen had no significant effect on joint degeneration, while diclofenac sodium and sulphinpyrazone (which has no anti-inflammatory properties) tended to delay it.

In a separate nine-month study, diclofenac sodium reduced both the incidence and the severity of lesions, while indomethacin had the opposite effects. These beneficial actions of diclofenac sodium should be attributed not to potential anti-arthrotic activity but to sparing of connective tissue.

In man, the progression of primary osteoarthrosis (OA) is slow and difficult to assess. Also, therapeutic effects of pharmacological agents are not readily evident in this condition, and prolonged observation is necessary to detect them. To circumvent these problems, a great variety of experimental models of induced OA in rats, rabbits, chickens and dogs are in use. In some, pathological changes are evoked by the application of mechanical forces, for example, constant pressure (Salter and Field, 1960), or single or repeated jolts to the joints (Radin and Paul, 1971), by induction of the valgus position (Columbo *et al.*, 1983; Liebig and Weseloh, 1979), or by amputation of the forelegs (Kanie *et al.*, 1979), bringing about traumatic impaction. Changes in the articular cartilage eventually leading to destruction are also elicited by over-use or under-use of the joints (Wilhelmi and Maier, 1983) or immobilisation (Videman *et al.*, 1977). The disease can also be provoked by administration of non-physiological materials, such as iodo-acetate (Kalbhen and Blum, 1977), or even of physiological substances such as vitamin A (Lenzi *et al.*, 1974), proteolytic enzymes (Bentley, 1974), cartilage homogenate (Caruso *et al.*, 1968) and blood (haemarthrosis) (Pad Bosch and Putte, 1979). The most frequent means of induction, however, is surgery. The wide range of operative interventions performed also includes scarification of the articular cartilage, removal of condyle, of either the femur or tibia, partial or total transection of the cruciate ligaments, and displacement or removal of the patella. Most of these operations produce a rapid deterioration of the cartilage, which is, under these conditions, hardly susceptible at all to the influence of drugs.

In contrast to these many models of induced OA, spontaneous occurrence of the disease has only been described in a few animal strains suitable for experimental studies, although spontaneous OA is a common disease observed in almost any animal species. These observations are largely due to the fundamental work of the Silberbergs and of Sokoloff. They identified an idiopathic, metabolic or age-dependent OA in guinea-pigs (Sokoloff, 1959), in mice of the YBR/Wi strain (Silberberg and Silberberg, 1956), and in C57 black mice (Silberberg, 1971; Sokoloff, 1956). The mouse strain STR/1N (Silberberg, 1971) or STR/ORT (Walton, 1977) and also the dogs used by Lust and Miller (1977) show obvious anatomical anomalies (displacement of the patella, laxity of ligaments) responsible for the development of OA.

Since we are concerned chiefly with the aetiopathogenesis of OA and assessment of the effects of drugs, we have opted for the spontaneous-disease model in the C57 black mouse.

CHARACTERISATION OF THE DISEASE

The development of the disease in the C57 black mouse is demonstrated in the accompanying series of histological sections. Figure 1 shows normal cartilage in a healthy young mouse, stained for proteoglycans with alcian blue. The dense packing of chondrocytes is typical of normal mouse cartilage. An initial manifestation of incipient disease is loss of staining and rarefaction of chondrocytes in the middle and deeper part of the cartilage (Fig. 2). Surface damage and vertical fissures (Fig. 3) occur thereafter. In some of the animals, a horizontal rupture along the 'tide-mark' is a first sign of damage, although the surface appears uninjured (Fig. 4). This horizontal tear might arise as a consequence of excessive water uptake occurring during the

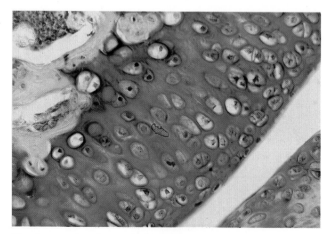

Fig. 1. Normal cartilage in a healthy young mouse, stained for proteoglycans with alcian blue. Chondrocytes densely packed—a typical finding.

early stages of cartilage destruction. As shown in Fig. 5, a whole portion becomes detached, possibly due to mechanical stresses during locomotion.

The loose particle of detritus eventually comes into contact with the synovial membrane (Fig. 6), which then engulfs and digests it. During this process, particularly when the shed material is excessive, an inflammatory reaction ensues, leading to synovitis (Fig. 7) with all its consequences, such as pain, release of proteolytic enzyme, tissue proliferation, pannus formation, and so on. The exposed calcified cartilage is quickly worn down to the underlying bone (Fig. 8). During this process of cartilage destruction, the subchondral bone becomes sclerotic, and the size of the bone-marrow cavities drastically reduced. Eventually, the underlying bone is abraded as well (Fig. 9). It is of interest to note that in this model the tibia is always worse affected than the femur.

In addition to the destructive processes, attempts at repair have been observed. Out of the junction between the cartilage and the synovial membrane emerges newly formed tissue, which takes stain for proteoglycans and contains cells resembling chondrocytes in appearance (Fig. 10), and which moves in the direction of the lesion. Unfortunately, the new tissue undergoes changes mainly before reaching the denuded bone. Chondrocyte clusters are formed and the tissue, essentially the matrix, loses its stainability for proteoglycans (Figs 11 and 12). We consider the formation of chondrocyte clusters to be an indication of a more or less ineffectual regenerative process. In mice, as in other species, including man, osteophytes are formed (Fig. 13).

The earliest manifestations of cartilage lesions were found in mice aged six months. The progression of the disease is linear throughout the animals' life-span of about two years (Fig. 14). At the age of 16–18 months, as many as 80% of the animals can be affected. The remaining 20% seem to be free of OA. It has been suggested that the severity of the disease is directly proportional to malposition of the hind legs, measured in terms of deviation from the axis (Draenert, personal communication). The unaffected animals display no malposition.

The progression of the disease is much slower in C57 black

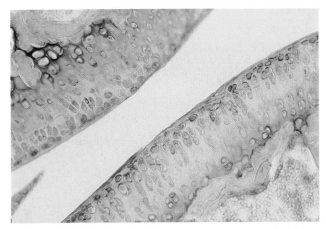

Fig. 2. Incipient OA in the mouse model: lack of staining and rarefaction of chondrocytes in central and deeper zones of the cartilage.

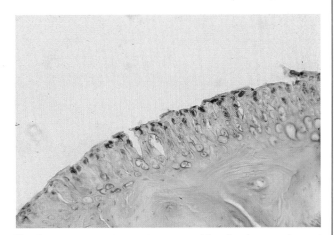

Fig. 3. Early changes of OA in the mouse model: surface damage and vertical fissuring.

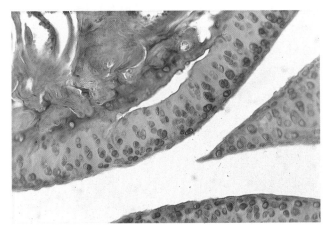

Fig. 4. Horizontal rupture at the cartilage 'tide-mark', without surface damage, is also seen as an early change.

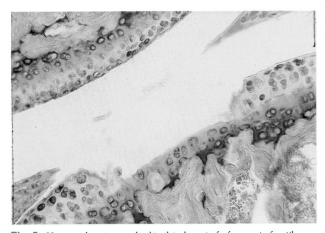

Fig. 5. Horizontal rupture can lead to detachment of a fragment of cartilage.

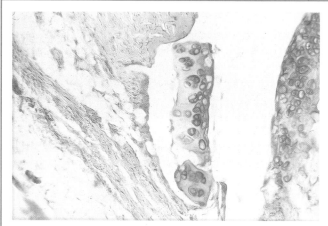

Fig. 6. Detritus mostly comes into contact with synovial membrane, which then engulfs and digests it.

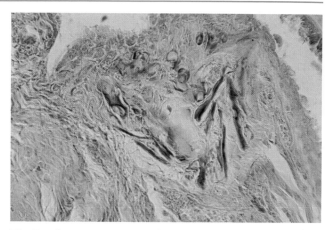

Fig. 7. Inflammatory reaction round ingested detritus: synovitis.

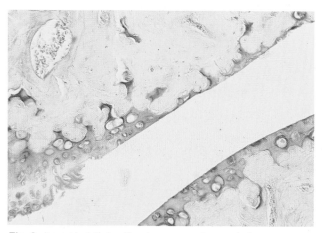

Fig. 8. Exposed calcified cartilage is soon worn down to the bone.

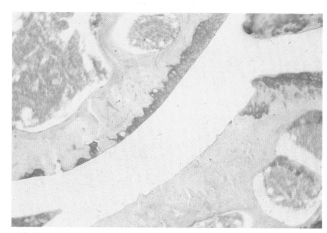

Fig. 9. Eventually the underlying bone is abraded as well.

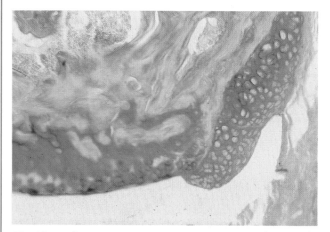

Fig. 10. Simultaneous attempts at repair: new tissue, staining for proteoglycans and containing chondrocyte-like cells, forms at the junction of synovium and cartilage.

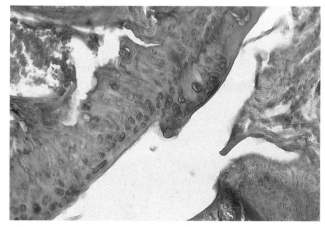

Fig. 11. The new tissue undergoes changes before reaching the denuded bone, losing stainability for proteoglycans, while the chondrocytes can form clusters.

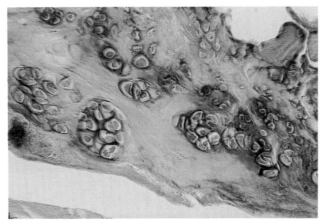

Fig. 12. Chondrocyte clusters under greater magnification. They represent a more or less ineffectual attempt at regeneration.

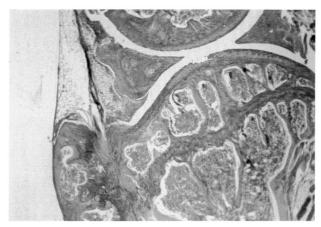

Fig. 13. Osteophyte formation.

mice than in STR/1N mice, and also in regular white laboratory mice from our own breeding unit (MAGf), and the effects of drugs are therefore more readily demonstrable.

METHODS

Except in a few experiments in which a solution is injected subcutaneously, the mice are treated by gavage, once daily five days a week, usually for four months. The knee joints are removed by severing the bones 1 cm above and below the articulation; they are then carefully freed of soft tissue, placed in a decalcifying solution, and embedded intact in paraffin blocks. This procedure avoids mechanical damage to the joints. From each knee joint, 50–100 sagittal sections 10 μm thick are cut by microtome. The sections are stained for proteoglycans with alcian blue and nuclear-fast red and inspected under the light microscope.

Two parameters are assessed. First, the incidence of lesions

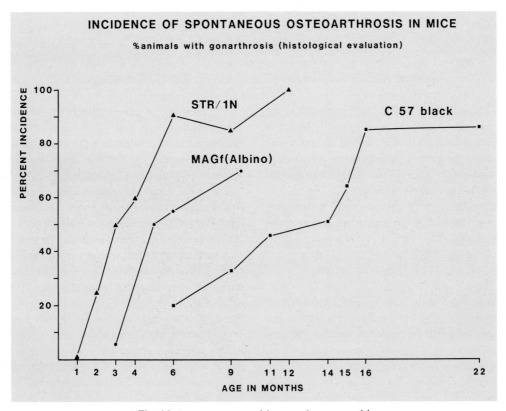

Fig. 14. Linear progression of disease in the mouse model.

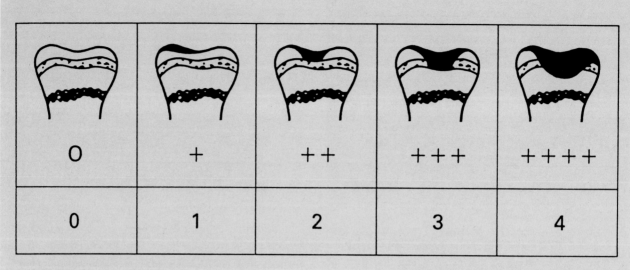

0	+	+ +	+ + +	+ + + +
0	1	2	3	4

O = Changes in the knee joint attributable to ageing only, with no definite evidence of osteoarthrosis; surface of the joint intact.

+ = Fissuring and fibrillation in the surface of the cartilage (collagenous fibres exposed); possibly cysts in the cartilage.

+ + = Small "punched out" defects or areas of abrasion in the non-calcified cartilage.

+ + + = Shallow defects extending into the calcified cartilage, but not into the bone itself; subchondral sclerosis.

+ + + + = Deep defects extending into the epiphyseal bone; eburnation of the subchondral bone; usually marginal proliferation of the joint cartilage.

Fig. 15. Arbitrary four-point scale for rating intensity of osteoarthrotic changes.

is determined by counting the affected joints, irrespective of the severity of the damage. Second, the severity of the lesions is rated on an arbitrary scale (Fig. 15): slight surface damage scores one plus; two plusses are given if cartilage is missing down to the 'tide-mark', three if all cartilage has been completely abraded in parts, and four if the bone is also affected.

Each treatment group, and the control group, is composed of some 25 mice at the start of the experiment and averages 19–21 animals at necropsy.

RESULTS

Two types of drug have been investigated: 'anti-arthrotics' reported to be potentially capable of modifying the disease; and analgesics with anti-inflammatory properties used for symptomatic relief.

The results are expressed as percentages of the corresponding control values for each experiment. Retardation of the degenerative process is considered to be an improvement, and its acceleration an aggravation of the disease.

The incidence of arthrotic joints tended to be less frequent after treatment with each of the anti-arthrotic drugs tested, except glucosamine sulphate in the smaller dose (Table I). Apart from glucosamine, the first four drugs are either extracted or synthetic polysulphated carbohydrates.

The two remaining drugs have venotropic properties. Rutoside showed marginal activity, but tribenoside, a hexose derivative with three substituent molecules of benzoic acid, reduced the incidence of affected joints significantly.

A very similar pattern emerges when the degrees of severity of the lesions are compared (Table I). Damage was less severe after treatment with all but two of the drugs. The slight negative effect of the polysulphated glycosaminoglycans (GAG) is indistinguishable from the controls, but the effect of the lower dose of glucosamine sulphate is marked.

The analgesics employed to alleviate pain during inflammatory episodes gave varying results with regard to incidence and severity of lesions (Table II). As expected, prednisone aggravated the disease in a dose-dependent fashion, but naproxen, ibuprofen, acetylsalicylic acid and phenylbutazone also

Table I. Effect of potential anti-arthrotic drugs on incidence and intensity of osteoarthrotic lesions in C57 black mice

Drug[a]	Daily dose[b] (mg/kg)	Treatment, months[b] (route of admin.)	Incidence of affected joints[c]	Intensity of osteo-arthrotic lesions[d]
PS GAG	5	2½ (s.c.)	− 8	+11
	15		− 8	+ 6
GAGP	0·1	2½ (s.c.)	−33	−43
	0·3		−21	−21
CHS	50	4 (p.o.)	−26	−14
	150		−26	−13
GAS	25	4 (p.o.)	+21	+52
	75		−12	+ 5
TRIB	30	3 (p.o.)	−43	−50
	100		−42	−41
	100	10 (p.o.)	−30	−18
	300		−26	−25
HER	30	3 (p.o.)	−19	− 5
	100		− 3	−18
	300		− 6	−10

[a]PS GAG, Polysulphated glycosaminoglycans (Arteparon®); GAGP, Cartilage, bone marrow extract (Rumalon®); CHS, Chondroitin sulphate (Structum®); GAS, Glucosamine sulphate (Dona 200®); TRIB, Tribenoside (Glyvenol®); HER, Hydroxy-ethyl-rutoside (Venoruton®).

[b]Administered daily five times a week.

[c]Number of affected joints expressed as a percentage of controls. Negative figures denote fewer and positive figures more affected joints than for untreated animals.

[d]Assessed by an arbitrary score, expressed as a percentage of controls. Plus indicates more and minus fewer extended lesions than for untreated mice.

accelerated the spontaneous progression of the disease. Indomethacin and pirprofen had no significant effect. Diclofenac sodium and sulphinpyrazone, a drug with no anti-inflammatory properties, slowed the rate of articular deterioration.

In a separate study, the effects of diclofenac sodium and indomethacin were compared after their administration once every other week for nine months. Diclofenac sodium reduced both incidence (Fig. 16) and severity of lesions, while indomethacin had the opposite effect.

DISCUSSION

The majority of the drugs reported to be potential anti-arthrotic agents retarded the progression of the disease to a varying extent. The most pronounced effect, which was statistically significant at the 5% level, or higher, was produced by tribenoside. The mode of action of these drugs is obscure, but it is noteworthy that they belong to widely differing therapeutic categories. Some of the polysulphated (poly)-saccharides have been shown to interfere with proteolytic enzymes (Baici and Fehr, 1980), but that could hardly be their sole effect. The hypothesis that they may serve as substrates for the biosynthesis of GAG

seems far-fetched and most unlikely, considering the small doses given. In patients, these preparations are administered in soluble form not eliciting synovitis as manifested by detrital particles. Repeated intra-articular injection of, for example, polysulphated GAG could eventually lead to haemarthrosis, through extravasation of blood from pierced capillaries into the joint space and emphasised by the anticoagulant properties of the drug.

The other anti-arthrotics tested have venotropic activity. It seems reasonable to assume that they act by improving the microcirculation, either in the synovial membrane or in the subchondral bone. Whether they improve the nutrition of cartilage or help to clear obstructions to the removal of degradation products remains to be seen. Despite the many questions still open, it is encouraging that seemingly beneficial drugs with differing modes of action were identified.

The drugs most widely prescribed at present for the treatment of OA are analgesics of the non-steroidal anti-inflammatory type. These compounds are reported to inhibit proteolytic enzymes (Kruze et al., 1976), but also interfere with proteoglycan synthesis, as measured by incorporation of sulphate (Boström et al., 1964). The two effects tend to cancel each other out; whether, or under what circumstances, one might prevail over the other in a particular drug cannot be predicted from their chemical structures. Granting this possibility, however, the disparities noted in the effects of the tested analgesics on articular cartilage would be less surprising.

Most of the drugs displayed a dose-dependent effect. The doses used were chosen on data from assays in animals of their

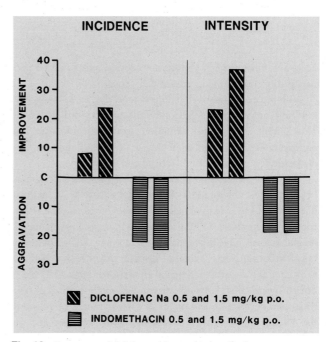

Fig. 16. Comparison of diclofenac sodium and indomethacin.

Table II. Effect of non-steroidal anti-inflammatory drugs on incidence and intensity of osteoarthrotic lesions in C57 black mice

Drug	Daily dose[ab] (mg/kg)	Treatment, months[b] (route of admin.)	Incidence of affected joints[c]	Intensity of osteoarthrotic lesions[d]
Prednisone	1	4 (p.o.)	+ 13	− 1
	3		+ 37	+ 11
	10		+178	+122
Naproxen	15	4 (p.o.)	− 10	+ 11
	50		+ 66	+ 48
Ibuprofen	15	4 (p.o.)	+ 10	+ 5
	50		+ 48	+ 68
Acetyl-salicylic acid	50	5 (p.o.)	+ 38	+ 53
	150		+ 40	+ 66
Phenyl-butazone	15	5 (p.o.)	+ 8	+ 8
	50		+ 25	+ 63
Indomethacin	1	4 (p.o.)	+ 12	+ 35
	3		+ 16	+ 19
Pirprofen	10	4 (p.o.)	− 11	− 10
	30		− 11	0
	100		0	− 11
Diclofenac sodium	0·3	4 (p.o.)	− 13	− 27
	1		− 14	− 24
	3		− 28	− 8
Sulphin-pyrazone	5	4 (p.o.)	+ 8	+ 3
	15		− 45	− 51
	50		− 21	− 14

[a]Dose chosen for equipotency of anti-inflammatory and analgesic efficacy in animals.
[b]Administered once daily except weekends.
[c]Number of affected joints expressed as a percentage of controls. Positive figures denote more and negative figures fewer affected joints than for untreated mice. The control mice displayed an incidence of 43–73% (average 56% of 10 collectives).
[d]Assessed by an arbitrary score, expressed as a percentage of controls. Plus indicates more and minus fewer extended lesions than for untreated mice.

acute anti-inflammatory and antinociceptive activity and do not necessarily correspond to human daily doses.

With the exception of sulphinpyrazone, the tested drugs possess both antinociceptive and anti-inflammatory properties and also inhibit prostanoid formation from arachidonate. Sulphinpyrazone is a chemical analogue of phenylbutazone; the diametrically opposite effects are difficult to explain.

The beneficial effect of diclofenac sodium, for instance, should be interpreted not as a sign of potential anti-arthrotic activity but rather of the absence of adverse effects on connective tissue. Clinical observations will show whether these findings in experimental animals have a bearing on OA in man. Like experimentally induced OA, murine disease admittedly has its shortcomings as an experimental model of human OA, but it does provide valuable insight into the aetiopathogenesis of arthrotic joint destruction and serves as a useful means of assessing the activity of drugs with disease-modifying capacity and the side effects of commonly prescribed analgesics.

REFERENCES

BAICI, A. and FEHR, K. (1980) Hemmung menschlicher lysosomaler Elastase durch Arteparon[R]. In: *Internationales Arzneimittel-Symposium Arteparon[R]*, IX European Congress of Rheumatology, Wiesbaden, 1979, N. Dettmer *et al.* (Eds), p. 19. Eular, Basle.

BENTLEY, G. (1974) Experimental osteoarthrosis. In: *Proceedings of the Symposium on Normal and Osteoarthrotic Articular Cartilage*, London, 1973, S.Y. Ali *et al.* (Eds), pp. 259–280. Institute of Orthopaedics, Stanmore.

BOSTRÖM, H., BERNTSEN, K. and WHITEHOUSE, M.W. (1964) Biochemical properties of anti-inflammatory drugs. II: Some effects on sulphate-^{35}S metabolism *in vivo*. *Biochem. Pharmacol.* **13**, 413–420.

CARUSO, I., MANTELLINI, P. and DOLCI, E. (1968) Modificazioni del PCS e CS della cartilagine indotte nel coniglio da un omogenato di cartilagine omologa. *Reumatismo* **20**(5), 420–426.

COLOMBO, C., BUTLER, M., O'BYRNE, E., HICKMAN, L., SWARTZEN-

DRUBER, D., SELWYN, M. and STEINETZ, B. (1983) A new model of osteoarthritis in rabbits: I. Development of knee joint pathology following lateral meniscectomy and section of the fibular collateral and sesamoid ligaments. *Arthritis Rheum.* **26**, 875–886.

KALBHEN, D.A. and BLUM, U. (1977) Experimental osteoarthrosis in hens. *Arzneimittelforsch.* **27/I**(3), 527–531.

KANIE, R., ABEMATSU, N., IMAIZUMI, T., KAMATA, S., OHTA, H. and MAEDA, M. (1979) Pathogenesis of osteoarthritis seen linked to overloading stress, postural changes. In: *Proc. 14th Cong. Int. Chir. Orthop. Traumatol.*, Kyoto.

KRUZE, D., FEHR, K., MENNINGER, R. and BÖNI, A. (1976) Effect of antirheumatic drugs on neutral proteases from human leucocyte granules. *Z. Rheumatol.* **35**, 337–346.

LENZI, L., BERLANDA, P., FLORA, A., AURELI, G., RIZZOTTI, M., BALDUINI, C. and BONI, M. (1974) Vitamin A-induced osteoarthritis in rabbits: an experimental model for the study of human disease. In: *Proceedings of the Symposium on Normal and Osteoarthrotic Articular Cartilage*, London, 1973, S.Y. Ali *et al.* (Eds), pp. 243–257. Institute of Orthopaedics, Stanmore.

LIEBIG, K. and WESELOH, G. (1979) Medikamentöse Beeinflussung bei experimentell erzeugter Arthrose. *66. Tagung Deutsch. Ges. Orthop. Traumatol.*, Basle, p. 51. Abstract.

LUST, G. and MILLER, D.R. (1977) Metabolic changes in cartilage from young dogs with degenerative joint disease. In: *AR/Heberden Society: International Symposium on the Aetiopathogenesis of Osteoarthrosis*, Cardiff.

PAD BOSCH, P.J.I.VAN 't and VAN DER PUTTE, L.B.A. (1979) Sequential radiological changes in rat knee joints during experimental chronic hemarthrosis. IX European Congress of Rheumatology, Wiesbaden, 1979. Abstract 140.

RADIN, E.L. and PAUL, I.L. (1971) The role of subchondral bone in the etiology of primary osteoarthrosis. In: *7th European Congress on Rheumatology*, Brighton. Abstract No. 36.11.

SALTER, R.B. and FIELD, P. (1960) The effects of continuous compression on living articular cartilage. *J. Bone Joint Surg.* **42**A, 31–49.

SILBERBERG, M. and SILBERBERG, R. (1956) Faulty skeletal development in 'yellow' mice. *Anat. Rec.* **124**, 129–143.

SILBERBERG, R. (1971) Wachstum und Altern des Skeletts. Documenta Geigy, *Acta rheumatol.* **26**.

SOKOLOFF, L. (1956) Pathologic anatomy of degenerative joint disease in mice. *A.M.A. Arch. Pathol.* **62**, 118–128.

SOKOLOFF, L. (1959) Osteoarthritis in laboratory animals. *Lab. Invest.* **8**, 1209–1217.

VIDEMAN, T., MICHELSSON, J.E. and LANGESKIÖLD, A. (1977) The development of radiographic changes in experimental osteoarthrosis provoked by immobilisation of the knee in rabbits. *Med. Sci. Biomed. Tech.* **5**, 1–2.

WALTON, M. (1977) Degenerative joint disease in the mouse knee: histological observations. *J. Pathol.* **123**, 109–122.

WILHELMI, G. and MAIER, R. (1983) Experimentelle Untersuchungen zur Aetiopathogenese der Arthrose. *Kassenarzt* **16**, 38–48.

Chapter 7

Effect of Selected Antirheumatic Agents on Surgically-induced Degenerative Knee Joint Disease in Rabbits

B. G. STEINETZ*, C. COLOMBO, M. C. BUTLER, E. M. O'BYRNE,
L. Y. HICKMAN, J. J. CHART and D. C. SWARTZENDRUBER

Research Department, Pharmaceuticals Division, CIBA-GEIGY Corporation, Ardsley, New York, USA

*Now at Laboratory for Experimental Medicine and Surgery on Primates, New York University Medical Centre.

SUMMARY

The lesion brought about by joint instability following lateral meniscectomy in the rabbit has been used as a model for studying whether established antirheumatic drugs can retard or reverse the resulting cartilage degeneration.

Operated animals were given systemic or intra-articular injection of the test drugs at stated dosages, or placebo injections consisting of excipient only. After six weeks, animals were killed and samples of tibial and femoral cartilage taken for study. Lesions were scored by a defined method taking into account 11 categories of histological changes, the tissue slides being coded and read blind.

The most clearcut protection against cartilage destruction was afforded by the glucocorticoids paramethasone and triamcinolone; of the other drugs tested only tribenoside, tranexamic acid and pirprofen offered more than 50% protection.

Certain drugs thus retard the progression of surgically-induced osteoarthritis in rabbits, without correction of the joint instability. The mechanisms by which these drugs act are not known, but they may involve inhibition of synovial and/or meniscus factors, such as catabolins and/or chondrocyte-produced proteases.

INTRODUCTION

Therapeutic efforts in degenerative joint disease in human beings have been primarily directed towards relief of pain and swelling by means of non-steroidal drugs with anti-inflammatory and analgesic properties. There is no evidence that such drugs retard or reverse the cartilage-degrading processes which underlie the disease; indeed, there are suggestions that some of these drugs may actually have adverse effects on cartilage metabolism (Palmoski and Brandt, 1979, 1980, 1982; Palmoski et al., 1980).

A few years ago we became interested in the possibility of developing new test systems that might reveal unique chondroprotective or chondroregenerative properties of new chemical entities being synthesised for our antirheumatic drug programme (Steinetz et al., 1981). If successful, such methodology would provide significant additional preclinical information both for drug design and for potential therapeutic profile.

It seemed naive to believe that any of the animal models of spontaneous or induced osteoarthritis (OA) described in the literature would faithfully reproduce all aspects of the disease in man. However, it appeared likely that the final common pathway leading to breakdown of cartilage matrix components might be similar in the animal and human diseases. Therefore, we sought to develop an animal model that produced degenerative joint disease in a *predictable location* and within a reasonable *time frame*, thus permitting practical assessment of pharmacological agents.

Many laboratories have produced essentially similar pathological changes in articular cartilage using various surgical techniques to induce knee-joint instability in rabbits or dogs: these include section of various supportive ligaments, partial or complete meniscectomy, or a combination of these procedures (for recent reviews see Schwartz and Greenwald, 1980; Steinetz et al., 1981; Hulth, 1982; Troyer, 1982).

Meniscectomy was attractive for the following reasons:

1. The incidence of the induced disease is virtually 100%
2. Cartilage lesions appear within a reasonable time frame
3. Lesions appear in a predictable location
4. The disease is similar in aetiology and pathogenesis to the secondary OA which frequently occurs in human beings as a consequence of meniscectomy (see, for example, Jones et al., 1978).

The detailed procedure for lateral partial meniscectomy with section of the fibular collateral and sesamoid ligaments in rabbits is described in detail elsewhere (Colombo et al., 1983a and b).

Our objectives in this study were to determine:

1. If pharmacological intervention in knee cartilage degradation is possible without correcting the joint instability
2. What types of known drugs might retard or reverse cartilage degeneration
3. The mechanisms by which drugs might intervene in the degenerative process
4. The relevance of such data to OA in human beings.

We have achieved our first two objectives but considerably more work will be required to complete the others. This paper therefore constitutes a progress report on our findings to date.

MATERIALS AND METHODS

Adult male New Zealand rabbits weighing approximately 4 kg were subjected to partial lateral meniscectomy and section of the fibular collateral and sesamoid ligaments of the right knee, as previously described (Colombo et al., 1983a).

Unless otherwise specified, drugs were administered either systemically five days a week for five weeks from the first to the sixth week after surgery or intra-articularly (i.a.) as two injections one and two weeks after surgery. Surgical controls received the appropriate vehicles. The rabbits were killed at the end of the sixth week after surgery and tibial and femoral cartilages were sampled, fixed, sectioned and stained for histological study exactly as described previously (Colombo et al., 1983a). The finished slides were coded and read blind. Individual lesions were scored for severity as shown in Table I. The lesion scores were used in two ways: *lesion profiles* were constructed to indicate how each drug influences the incidence and severity of individual lesion types; *total lesion scores* for tibial and femoral cartilage were calculated and used for statistical analysis by the Wilcoxon rank sum method (Colombo et al., 1983a and b; Butler et al., 1983).

Table I. Parameters evaluated 'blind' in tibial and femoral cartilage

Articular cartilage abnormalities	+1	+2	Scores +3	+4
Loss of superficial layer	Slight	Moderate	Focally severe	Extensively severe
Ulceration or erosion	Detectable	Moderate	Focally severe	Extensively severe
Fibrillation (surface fragmentation)	Noticeable	Moderate	Marked	Extensive
Fissures (V-shaped clefts)	1 very small	1 small	2 small or 1 medium	2 small, 2 medium or 1 large
Cysts	1 very small	1 small	2 small or 1 large	3 small or 2 large
Osteophytes/chondrophytes	Very small	Small	Medium	Large
Loss of stainable proteoglycan (safraninophilia)	Stain paler than control	Moderate loss	Marked loss	Total loss
Disorganisation of chondrocytes	Noticeable	Moderate, with some loss of columns	Marked loss of columns	No recognisable organisation
Clones	3–4 small[a] or 1–2 medium[b]	5–6 small or 3–4 medium or 1–2 large[c]	⩾ 7 small or 5–6 medium or 3–4 large	⩾ 7 medium or 5–6 large
Loss of chondrocytes	Noticeable	Moderate	Marked	Very extensive
Exposure of subchondral bone	Focal	Moderate	Fairly extensive	Very extensive

[a]Small = 2–4 cells.
[b]Medium = 5–8 cells.
[c]Large = 9 or more cells.
Data reproduced with permission from Colombo et al., 1983.

RESULTS AND DISCUSSION

The drugs tested, the doses administered, the numbers of control and treated rabbits and the means and ranges of the combined lesion scores are shown in Tables II and III. The most clearcut protection against cartilage degradation was afforded by the glucocorticoids, paramethasone acetate (72%) and triamcinolone (66%) administered orally (Table II), or triamcinolone hexacetonide (65%) given as a single i.a. injection (Table III). The only other drugs to offer more than 50% protection were tribenoside (54 and 65% at 100 and 200 mg/kg by mouth, Table II), tranexamic acid (64% at 5 mg i.a. × 2, Table III), and pirprofen (56% at 50 mg/kg by mouth, Table II).

Other drugs which may have exerted marginal effects on the progress of surgically-induced OA in rabbits were D-penicillamine, gold sodium thiomalate, and tamoxifen citrate (38–40%, Table II). With the exception of tamoxifen citrate (40%, $P < 0.005$), the differences between the lesion values for rabbits treated with penicillamine or gold and their corresponding controls were of only borderline significance ($P = 0.05$). Also, only the tibial or the femoral lesions, but not both, differed from controls in these groups, whereas scores for both tibial and femoral lesions were significantly lower in the rabbits treated with tamoxifen or with the more highly active drugs (i.e. steroids, tribenoside, tranexamic acid and pirprofen). Fur-

thermore, higher doses of penicillamine or gold resulted in insignificant changes in lesion scores. Thus these agents can only be regarded as questionably active in this assay. Similarly, a 14% reduction in lesion severity of benoxaprofen-treated rabbits was statistically significant ($P < 0.025$, Table II) but this appeared to be due to low femoral lesion scores in the treated animals and a very tight grouping in those of control animals. Since the apparent error in a subjective scoring system of 1–4 such as we use could easily be as high as $\pm 25\%$ and the mean score for benoxaprofen (48) falls within those of our historical control groups (33–57), we have to question the *biological* significance of these results. The benoxaprofen experiment has been included here to illustrate the need for common sense and scientific judgement when dealing with subjective data of this type.

The distribution of total lesion scores of individual rabbits treated with the more active compounds was compared with that of the respective surgical controls (Fig. 1). It is apparent that such treatment was associated with a shift in the lesion scores to the left (i.e. towards a lower severity) relative to those of the corresponding control animals. A basic assumption in the use of the Wilcoxon rank sum method of statistical analysis is that the two randomly selected groups of rabbits (treated and control) had the same potential for lesion development at the start of the experiment and would have exhibited a very similar distribution of lesion scores at the end of the experiment had

Table II. Drugs tested for systemic effects on surgically-induced osteoarthritis in rabbits

Compound type[a]	Generic name	Dose[a] mg/kg	No. of rabbits Control/ Treated	Mean combined lesion scores Control (range)	Drug (range)	% Inhibition	P
SAID[b]							
	Paramethasone acetate	0·1	8/7	50 (40–61)	14 (5–27)	72	<0·001
	Triamcinolone	0·1	4/4	48 (41–53)	16 (3–34)	66	<0·01
NSAID[c]							
	Indomethacin	1	4/3	56 (53–61)	47 (32–64)		n.s.
		10	6/5	52 (33–66)	33 (1–56)		n.s.
	Phenylbutazone	100	4/4	50 (48–54)	38 (19–51)		n.s.
	Benoxaprofen	25	8/7	56 (40–65)	48 (35–58)	14	<0·025
	Ibuprofen	30	4/4	50 (48–54)	52 (34–62)		n.s.
	Pirprofen	50	7/8	57 (34–85)	29 (3–65)	56	<0·02
	Piroxicam	25	8/8	56 (40–65)	49 (26–64)		n.s.
	Sodium salicylate	200	4/3	56 (53–61)	50 (40–61)		n.s.
	Tolmetin	10	8/7	47 (29–65)	34 (7–73)		n.s.
DMARD[d]							
	Chloroquine diphosphate	10	8/8	47 (24–61)	49 (32–58)		n.s.
		25	6/7	55 (31–69)	38 (23–67)		n.s.
	D-penicillamine HCl	25	7/8	48 (28–61)	30 (1–49)	38	=0·05
		50	8/7	42 (18–55)	28 (4–54)		n.s.
	Gold-Na thiomalate	3 i.m.	8/8	48 (28–61)	29 (4–67)	40	=0·05
		6 i.m.	8/8	42 (18–55)	37 (10–56)		n.s.
	Auranofin	5	8/7	33 (3–54)	31 (14–55)		n.s.
Miscellaneous							
	Orgotein	0·5 s.c.	9/8	52 (28–77)	34 (6–62)		n.s.
	Diacetylrhein	5	16/15	34 (3–54)	31 (15–49)		n.s.
	Tamoxifen citrate	0·5	8/8	50 (23–64)	30 (13–41)	40	<0·005
	Tribenoside	100	7/7	57 (34–85)	26 (9–65)	54	<0·01
		200	7/4	57 (34–85)	20 (5–30)	65	<0·025

[a]Unless otherwise specified—doses were administered by mouth 5 days per week for 5 weeks.
[b]Steroidal anti-inflammatory drug.
[c]Non-steroidal anti-inflammatory drug.
[d]Disease-modifying anti-rheumatic drug.
Data reproduced with permission from Colombo *et al.*, 1983.

an ineffective drug (or no drug) been given. An efficacious drug will lower the lesion scores of the treated group as a whole, but there will still be a range of values from least to most severe. In the case of paramethasone acetate the scores for the treated population fall entirely below those of the controls (Fig. 1). In the case of the other very effective drugs there was some overlap of scores of treated rabbits with those of the control group, although there was always a clear shift to the left (i.e. toward lowered severity) of the treated population relative to the controls (Fig. 1). It is obvious, however, that the histological changes in tibial and femoral cartilage which are the basis of the lesion scores may be indistinguishable in the overlapping animals of treated and control groups. The exception to this statement occurs when a drug may significantly affect only one or a few of the parameters. Accordingly, we have constructed lesion profiles for each of the drugs tested and compared these with the lesion profiles of control animals in each experiment. Lesion pro-

files for the active drugs shown in Fig. 1 are illustrated in Figs 2–6. It is apparent that the glucocorticoids paramethasone acetate (orally) and triamcinolone hexacetonide (i.a.) reduce the incidence and severity of most of the lesions under study (Figs 2 and 3). The most marked effects were to preserve cellular integrity, suppress osteophyte formation and prevent the more serious matrix abnormalities such as ulceration and fissuring. Tribenoside treatment likewise was associated with preservation of cellular architecture, suppression of osteophytes and a reduction in matrix abnormalities (Fig. 4). The profile for pirprofen (Fig. 5) was in general similar to that of tribenoside, while that for tranexamic acid showed not only a preservation of cellular architecture and a reduction in surface lesions but a remarkable reduction in the incidence and severity of proteoglycan loss in the femoral cartilage (Fig. 6).

Photomicrographs illustrating some typical protective effects of paramethasone acetate, tribenoside and tranexamic acid are

Table III. Drugs tested by intra-articular injection against surgically-induced osteoarthritis in rabbits

Compound type[a]	Generic name	Dose[a] mg × 2 (i.a.)[b]	No. of rabbits Control/ Treated	Mean combined lesion scores		% Inhibition	P
				Control (range)	Drug (range)		
SAID							
	Triamcinolone hexacetonide	1	9/10	51 (31–69)	18 (6–37)	65	<0·005
	Carbenoxolone Na	5	4/4	38 (29–50)	32 (22–50)		n.s.
	Algestone acetophenide	2	4/4	58 (36–77)	72 (58–77)		n.s.
NSAID							
	Phenylbutazone	25	4/4	58 (36–77)	68 (47–83)		n.s.
	Pirprofen	5	4/3	45 (23–68)	37 (23–53)		n.s.
Antiproteases							
	Pentosan polysulphate	0·1	8/8	31 (22–39)	43 (19–60)		n.s.
		5	6/6	52 (34–65)	56 (50–65)		n.s.
	Arteparon	2·5	8/8	31 (22–39)	39 (24–57)		n.s.
	Aprotinin	500 units	3/3	45 (23–68)	48 (43–51)		n.s.
	Tranexamic acid	5	7/7	44 (29–67)	16 (3–47)	64	<0·005
Miscellaneous							
	Orgotein	2	4/4	58 (36–77)	56 (50–65)		n.s.

[a,b]Abbreviations as in Table II.
Two i.a. injections given 1 and 2 weeks after surgery except for triamcinolone hexacetonide which was injected once 1 week after surgery.
Data reproduced with permission from Butler *et al.*, 1983.

shown in Figs 7 and 8. The reader will realise from inspection of Fig. 1 that all treated animals were not similarly protected; indeed cartilage samples from a few were indistinguishable from those of the surgical controls. Reconstruction of the entire tibial and femoral cartilage samples of pirprofen-treated and surgical control rabbits are shown in Figs 9 and 10, together with the actual lesion scores for these samples (Table IV). Although the drug afforded only partial protection, the differences between the cartilage of the drug- and vehicle-treated animals is none the less striking.

The mechanisms by which drugs may intervene in the degenerative joint disease which follows surgical creation of a joint instability are by no means clear.

In previous studies (Colombo *et al.*, 1983a) we showed that cutting the synovium alone or the synovium and/or lateral ligaments was insufficient to initiate cartilage degradation. It was only when the lateral menisci were detached that significant pathological changes appeared in tibial cartilage. Minns and Muckle (1982) have shown that division of the lateral meniscus in rabbits markedly reduces its role in resisting medial-lateral shear forces during normal physiological loading. We found that injuring the lateral meniscus by means of three radial cuts in addition to its detachment resulted in significant femoral as well as tibial pathology. However, partial lateral meniscectomy resulted in the development of the most severe lesions (Colombo *et al.*, 1983a and b). We speculated that, in addition to the mechanical instability created by the operative procedures, the damaged tissues (meniscus and synovium) may produce cartilage-degrading substances (proteases and/or catabolins?) which act locally on the tibial and femoral cartilage. This speculation is consonant with the rapid loss of meniscal safraninophilia (three days after surgery), the rapid rise in the lysosomal marker enzyme acid phosphatase and the increased uptake of ^{67}Ga in both synovium and meniscus which occurs after the partial

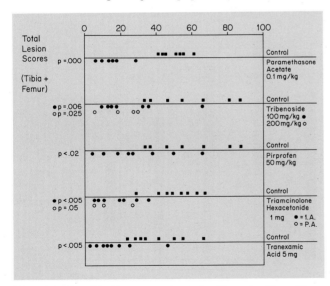

Fig. 1. Total combined lesion scores for tibial and femoral cartilage of knees of rabbits subjected to partial lateral meniscectomy and section of the fibular collateral and sesamoid ligaments: effects of different types of drug. Paramethasone acetate, tribenoside and pirprofen were administered orally five days a week from the first to the sixth week after surgery. Triamcinolone hexacetonide was injected i.a. or peri-articularly as a single dose one week after surgery. Tranexamic acid was injected i.a. seven and 14 days after surgery. Data reproduced with permission from Colombo *et al.* (1983b) and Butler *et al.* (1983).

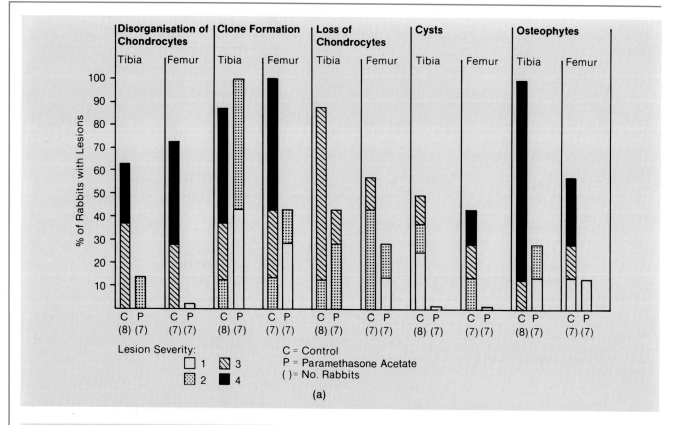

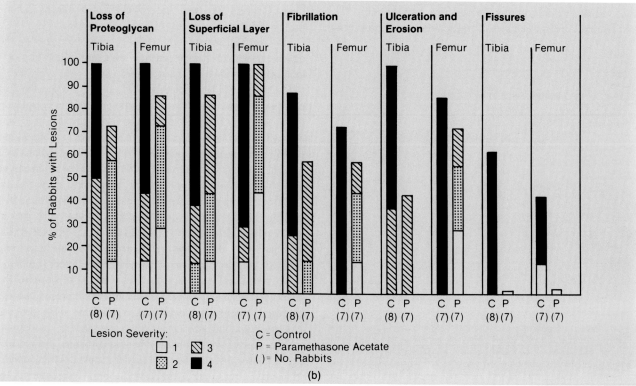

Fig. 2. Incidence and severity of abnormalities in tibial and femoral cartilage of surgical control rabbits and rabbits treated with paramethasone acetate. (a) Cellular abnormalities. (b) Matrix abnormalities. Reproduced with permission from Colombo *et al.* (1983b).

Table IV. Individual lesion scores for tibial and femoral cartilage samples shown in Figs 9 and 10

Tissue	Lesion	Sham control	Surgery control (OA)	Surgery plus pirprofen
Tibia (Fig. 9)	Loss of superficial layer	0	4	1
	Ulceration or erosion of cartilage	0	4	0
	Fibrillation	0	4	1
	Osteophytes	0	4	1
	Loss of proteoglycan	0	3	3
	Loss of cartilage	0	3	0
	Clones	0	4	2
	Exposure of bone	0	0	0
	Fissures	0	0	0
	Cysts	0	0	0
	Disorganisation of chondrocytes	0	2	2
	Loss of chondrocytes	0	3	1
	Total tibial score	0	31	11
Femur (Fig. 10)	Loss of superficial layer	0	4	1
	Ulceration or erosion of cartilage	0	3	0
	Fibrillation	0	4	1
	Osteophytes	0	0	0
	Loss of proteoglycan	0	3	3
	Loss of cartilage	0	3	0
	Clones	0	4	2
	Exposure of bone	0	0	0
	Fissures	0	4	0
	Cysts	0	0	0
	Disorganisation of chondrocytes	0	4	2
	Loss of chondrocytes	0	2	1
	Total femoral scores	0	31	10
	Total lesion score, tibia + femur	0	62	21

lateral meniscectomy (Colombo *et al.*, 1983a and b; Swartzendruber *et al.*, 1987). Histological changes in the synovium and meniscus are also suggestive of actively metabolising cells and a pannus-like tissue forms which invades the meniscus (Swartzendruber *et al.*, 1987). Similar hyperactive synovial tissues have also been described in a spontaneous model of OA in the dog (Lust and Wurster, 1987) and in earlier studies of primary OA or OA secondary to meniscectomy operations in human beings (see Muckle, 1982). Whether such synovial changes are a cause or a consequence of cartilage degeneration still remains unclear (Muckle, 1982).

Palmoski and Brandt (1982b) have recently shown that immobilisation by means of plaster casts prevents the development of OA secondary to section of the cruciate ligaments in knees of dogs. We need to do similar immobilisation experiments in rabbits with partial lateral meniscectomy and section of the lateral knee ligaments to determine the factors most involved in stimulating degenerative joint disease in this species. However, it is clearly inferred from the foregoing that any therapeutic drug effects observed in our own rabbit meniscectomy experiments would have to have been exerted on cellular and biochemical mechanisms of cartilage breakdown elicited by the surgical procedure itself (i.e. we made no effort to correct the joint instability *per se*). A similar conclusion can be reached regarding the numerous attempts at therapeutic intervention in degenerative joint disease in rabbits undertaken by Moskowitz and his colleagues (Moskowitz, 1977; Rosner *et al.*, 1979, 1980, 1981) and by Telhag (1973) who likewise did not correct the

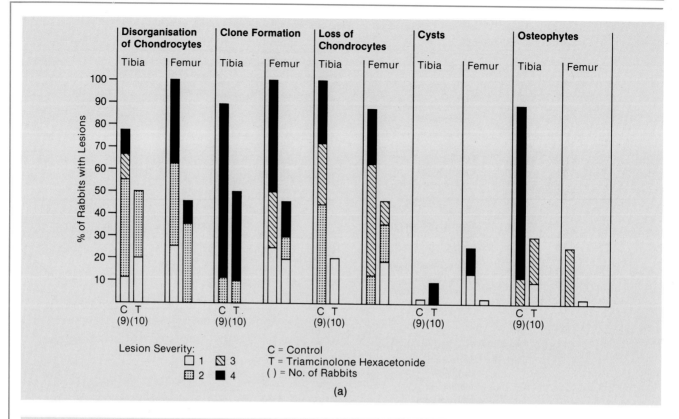

(a)

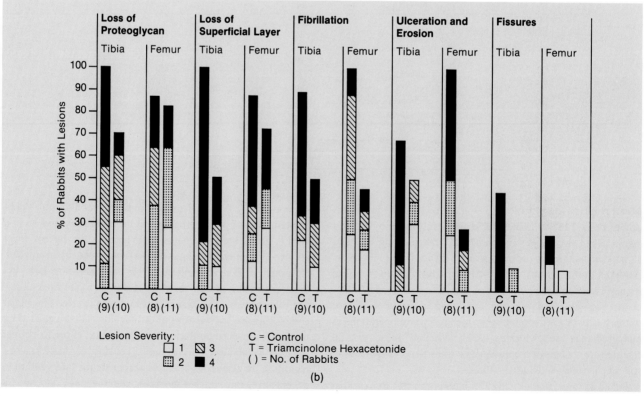

(b)

Fig. 3. Incidence and severity of abnormalities in tibial and femoral cartilage of surgical control rabbits and rabbits treated with triamcinolone hexacetonide. (a) Cellular abnormalities. (b) Matrix abnormalities.

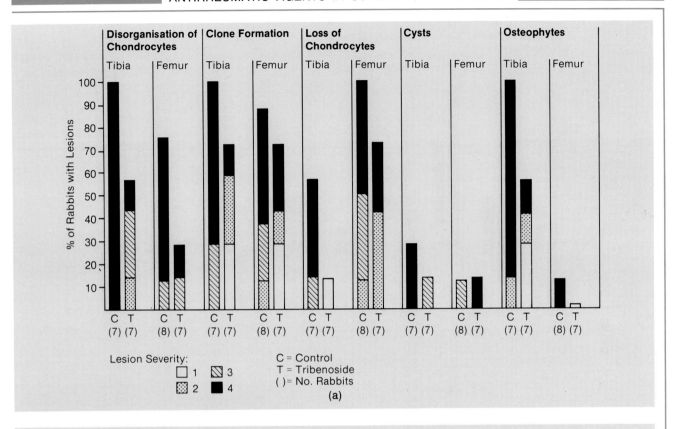

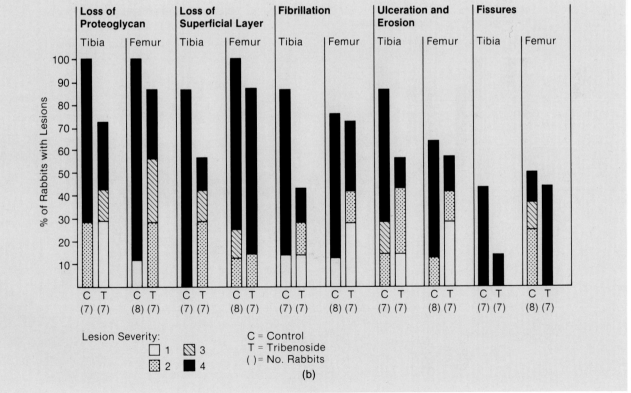

Fig. 4. Incidence and severity of abnormalities in knees of surgical control rabbits and rabbits treated with tribenoside. (a) Cellular abnormalities. (b) Matrix abnormalities.

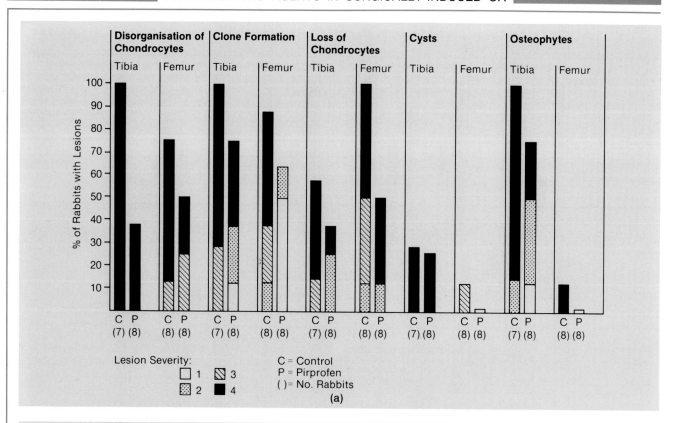

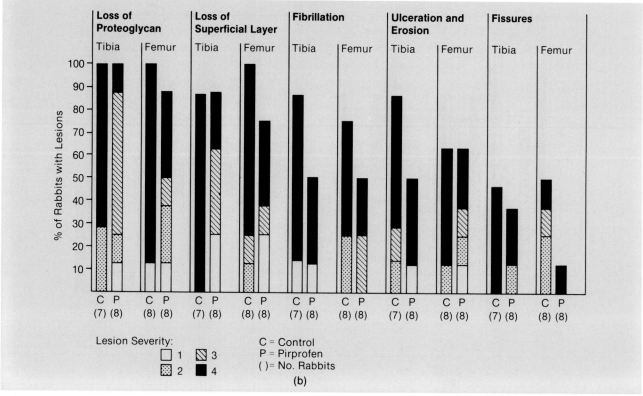

Fig. 5. Incidence and severity of abnormalities in knees of surgical control rabbits and rabbits treated with pirprofen. (a) Cellular abnormalities. (b) Matrix abnormalities.

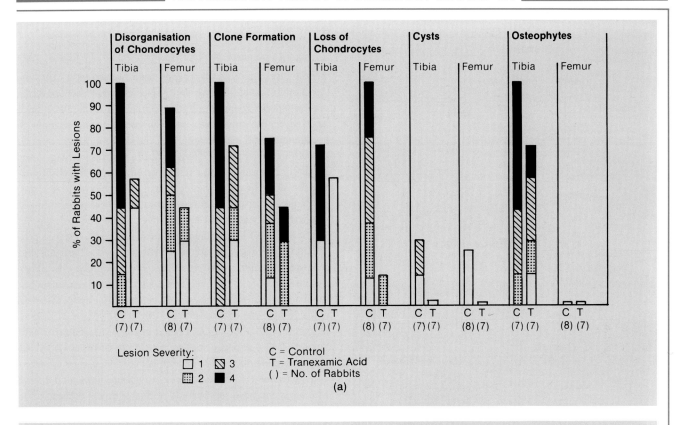

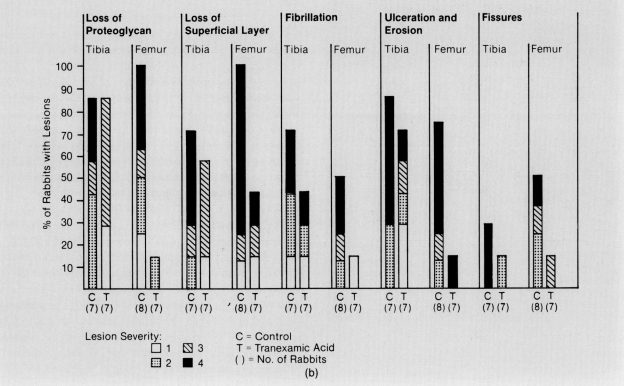

Fig. 6. Incidence and severity of abnormalities in tibial and femoral cartilage of surgical control rabbits and rabbits treated with tranexamic acid. (a) Cellular abnormalities. (b) Matrix abnormalities. Reproduced with permission from Butler *et al.* (1983).

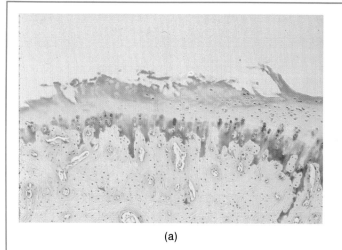

(a)

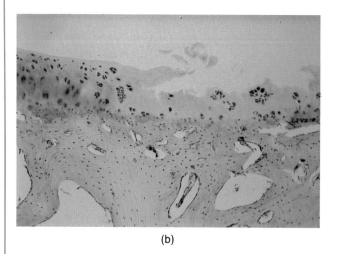

(b)

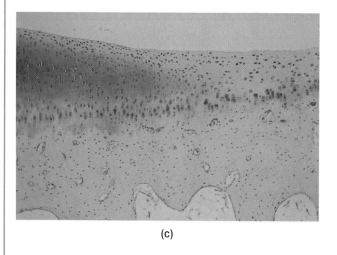

(c)

Fig. 7. Tibial cartilage lesions in rabbit knees six weeks after lateral meniscectomy. (a) Unoperated knee. (b) Operated knee. (c) Operated knee of a rabbit treated with triamcinolone hexacetonide, 1 mg i.a. one week after surgery. Safranin 0; × 150.

mechanical knee instability induced by their operative procedures.

Granted that the surgically-induced knee instability would persist throughout the experiments performed by the Moskowitz group, Telhag and ourselves, what then could be the targets for chemoprophylaxis? Stephens *et al.* (1979) have pointed to the similarities between osteoarthritic changes in spontaneous and experimental OA and the re-initiation of bone growth in the epiphysis. They postulate that the cartilage loses its ability to produce anti-angiogenic substances, thereby opening the door to an unwanted ingrowth of blood vessels and consequent destruction of articular cartilage and resumption of ossification processes. An equally attractive hypothesis suggests that trauma to the synovium and meniscus could result in production of cartilage-degrading proteases as well as synovial (and meniscal?) catabolin*-like mediators which stimulate the chondrocytes to produce the enzymes which destroy their surrounding matrix. Our own recent studies, reported elsewhere (Steinetz *et al.*, 1984, 1985; Schroder *et al.*, 1984; O'Byrne *et al.*, 1984), as well as those of others (Wood *et al.*, 1983; Sabiston and Adams, 1985), strongly suggest that synovial tissues obtained from osteoarthritic joints (experimentally induced or spontaneous) produce greater quantities of catabolin/interleukin-1-type mediators and proteases than do normal synovial tissues. In the case of lateral partial meniscectomy in rabbits, the synovial tissue from the operated knee shows increased metabolic activity in terms of increased synoviocyte labelling with tritiated thymidine, increased production of cathepsin B and increased production of catabolin in tissue culture as early as 1–2 weeks after surgery (Steinetz *et al.*, 1984, 1985; Schroder *et al.*, 1984).

Both the angiogenesis and synovial mediator hypotheses have merit; however, in surgically-induced OA in rabbits we would suggest that the synovial/meniscal factors may initiate cartilage degradation and account for proteoglycan loss, water inhibition and irregularities in the articular surfaces. These changes may then lead to further metabolic abnormalities in the chondrocytes themselves, which ultimately lead to loss of protection against capillary ingrowth, loss of chondrocytes, and re-initiation of bone growth (osteophyte formation).

The pharmacological profile of the drugs which exhibited activity in our model, as well as those of the Moskowitz group and Telhag, tend to support this latter interpretation. Both we and Moskowitz have found that glucocorticoids inhibit the progression of OA in rabbits (Moskowitz, 1977; Colombo *et al.*, 1983a and b). The mechanisms of their anti-OA effects may well be related to their ability to inhibit release and/or action of proteoglycanases, to stimulate the synthesis of enzyme inhibitors, to stabilise lysosomal enzymes and to inhibit release of catabolin-like factors (Steinberg *et al.*, 1979; Flower and Black-

---

*Catabolin is synonymous with interleukin-1.

96

well, 1979; Hill, 1981; Panagides *et al.*, 1980; Dingle, 1978, 1981; Stephens *et al.*, 1979). Glucocorticoids may also increase the strength of connective tissues by stabilising fibrillar aggregates of collagen molecules or increasing collagen crosslinking (Oxlund *et al.*, 1981; Steinetz *et al.*, 1966). It appears that classical anti-inflammatory activity *per se* has little to do with the actions observed with the glucocorticoids since other anti-inflammatory steroids (algestone acetophenide and carbenoxolone) were inactive, as were all but one of the non-steroidal anti-inflammatory drugs (NSAIDs) tested.

Telhag (1973) observed that tranexamic acid prevented proteoglycan loss (determined biochemically) from knee cartilage of medially meniscectomised rabbits, and we found that it inhibited the loss of histochemical safraninophilic staining of proteoglycan and prevented surface irregularities and cellular abnormalities. Tranexamic acid is a potent inhibitor of plasminogen activator and thus may protect both cartilage proteoglycan and collagen (plasmin is a potent proteoglycanase and also activates latent collagenase; Stephens *et al.*, 1979).

The mechanism of action of tribenoside in our model is completely unknown. However, we tested this drug because of a report that it retarded spontaneous degenerative joint disease in C57 B1 mice (Wilhelmi and Faust, 1976). This compound is a glucofuranoside derivative and as such may become involved (in some totally unknown way) in glycosaminoglycan metabolism or serve as a false substrate for proteoglycan-degrading enzymes. It is noteworthy that tribenoside is quite active in inhibiting proteoglycan breakdown in our *in vitro* synovium-cartilage co-culture model (O'Byrne *et al.*, 1987).

The mechanism whereby pirprofen retarded the development of OA-like lesions in our model is likewise obscure. It would appear not to be related to its anti-inflammatory activity, as all other 'profens'—indeed, all other NSAIDs tested—did not show significant activity. Pirprofen and another experimental drug found active in the lateral meniscectomy model, CGS 5391B (Colombo *et al.*, 1983b), were subsequently found to inhibit the lipoxygenase as well as the cyclooxygenase pathways of arachidonic acid metabolism, and an influence on the development of OA-like lesions via this pathway cannot be ruled out.

The marginally significant ($P = 0.05$) chondroprotective effects seen with the disease-modifying antirheumatic drugs (DMARDs) penicillamine and gold require further study. However, rabbits treated with increased doses of both of these compounds failed to show significant reduction in lesion scores.

Tamoxifen citrate, an anti-oestrogen, exhibited significant protection against lesion formation in our rabbit model and that of Rosner *et al.* (1981). It is doubtful whether this activity is related to anti-oestrogenic properties *per se*, inasmuch as we used adult male rabbits whereas Rosner *et al.* (1981) used immature females. Our own laboratories have shown that tamoxifen citrate binds to corticosteroid receptors and it is conceivable that the drug acts as a weak glucocorticoid.

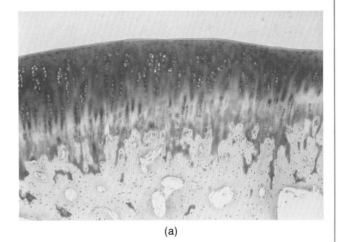

(a)

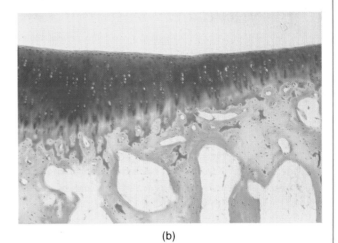

(b)

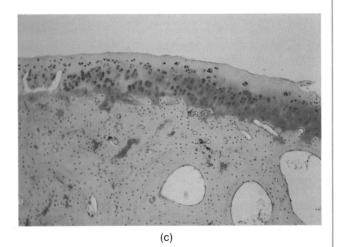

(c)

Fig. 8. Femoral cartilage lesions in rabbit knees six weeks after lateral meniscectomy. (a) Unoperated knee. (b) Operated knee. (c) Operated knee of a rabbit treated with triamcinolone hexacetonide, 1 mg i.a. one week after surgery. Safranin 0; × 150.

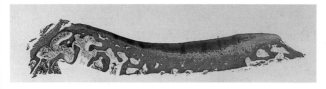
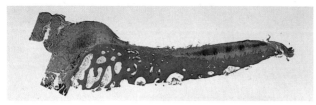
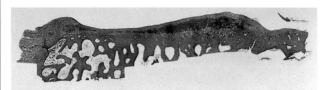

Fig. 9. Reconstructions of tissue sections of tibial cartilage from knees of rabbits which had undergone lateral meniscectomy. Top: sham-operated control. Middle: rabbit after lateral meniscectomy. Bottom: rabbit after lateral meniscectomy, treated with pirprofen (50 mg/kg by mouth five days/week for five weeks). Safranin 0; approximately × 30.

It is important to mention that Howell *et al.* (1985) reported that Arteparon®, a sulphated polysaccharide product known to be a protease inhibitor, is both prophylactically and therapeutically active in the Moskowitz medial meniscectomy model of OA in rabbits. Administration of the substance intra-articularly twice a week for 11 weeks prevented or reversed the development of OA-like lesions, and this effect was associated with suppression of cartilage neutral proteases (Howell *et al.*, 1985). Arteparon was not active when administered intra-articularly one and two weeks after surgery in the Colombo rabbit model (Colombo *et al.*, 1983b). It is probable that the difference is due to our failure to administer the compound for a sufficient period of time, and that the lateral meniscectomy procedure results in development of more severe lesions than does the medial meniscectomy method of Moskowitz.

CONCLUSIONS

We conclude from our studies and those of others that it is possible to retard by means of drugs the progression of surgically-induced OA in rabbits without first correcting the joint instability. Different types of compounds such as glucocorticoids, sulphated polysaccharides, glucofuranosides and aminohexane carboxylic acids may be active, and there is no apparent correlation with their anti-inflammatory properties. The mechanisms of action whereby these compounds slow cartilage degeneration are unknown, but we postulate the inhibition of synovial and/or meniscal factors (e.g. catabolins), and/or chondrocyte-produced proteases may be involved.

The proof of relevance of our model to human degenerative joint disease will ultimately depend on the development of novel drugs that prove to be chemically useful in the treatment of OA. This in turn will depend upon improved clinical methodologies for much earlier identification of individuals with a high risk of developing OA, and for monitoring progression or regression of the disease.

ACKNOWLEDGEMENTS

The authors much appreciate the critical discussions of our work and useful suggestions made by Drs A.M. White, M.K. Jasani, S. Ciccolunghi, A. Pataki and R. Maier.

We thank Mrs A. Potanovic for her skilful preparation of the manuscript.

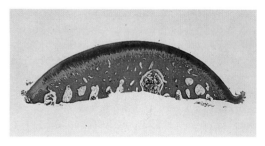
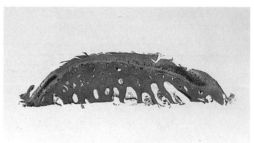
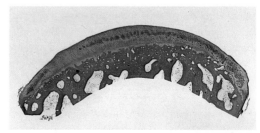

Fig. 10. Reconstructions of tissue sections of femoral cartilage from knees from rabbits which had undergone lateral meniscectomy. Top: sham-operated control. Middle: rabbit after lateral meniscectomy. Bottom: rabbit after lateral meniscectomy, treated with pirprofen as in Fig. 9. Safranin 0; approximately × 40.

REFERENCES

BUTLER, M., COLOMBO, C., HICKMAN, L., O'BYRNE, E., STEELE, R., STEINETZ, B., QUINTAVALLA, J. and YOKOYAMA, N. (1983) A new model of osteoarthritis in rabbits. III. Evaluation of anti-osteoarthritic effects of selected drugs administered intra-articularly. *Arthritis Rheum.* **26**, 1380–1386.

COLOMBO, C., BUTLER, M., HICKMAN, L., SELWYN, M., CHART, J. and STEINETZ, B. (1983b) A new model of osteoarthritis in rabbits: II. Evaluation of anti-osteoarthritic effects of selected antirheumatic drugs administered systemically. *Arthritis Rheum.* **26**, 1132–1139.

COLOMBO, C., BUTLER, M., O'BYRNE, E., HICKMAN, L., SWARTZEN-DRUBER, D., SELWYN, M. and STEINETZ, B. (1983a) A new model of osteoarthritis in rabbits: I. Development of knee joint pathology following lateral meniscectomy and section of the fibular collateral and sesamoid ligaments. *Arthritis Rheum.* **26**, 875–886.

DINGLE, J.T. (1978) Articular damage and its control. *Ann. Intern. Med.* **88**, 821–826.

DINGLE, J.T. (1981) Catabolin—a cartilage catabolic factor from synovium. *Clin. Orthop.* **156**, 219–231.

FLOWER, R. and BLACKWELL, G. (1979) Anti-inflammatory steroids induce biosynthesis of a phospholipase A_2 inhibitor which prevents prostaglandin generation. *Nature* **278**, 456–459.

HILL, D.J. (1981) Effects of cortisol on cell proliferation and proteoglycan synthesis and degradation in cartilage zones of the calf costochondral growth plate *in vitro* with and without rat plasma somatomedin activity. *J. Endocrinol.* **88**, 425–535.

HOWELL, D., MUNIZ, O. and CARRENO, M. (1985) The effect of glycosaminoglycan polysulfate ester (GAGPE) on proteoglycan degrading enzyme activity in an animal model of osteoarthritis (OA). In: *Proceedings of the Second International Conference of the Inflammation Research Association,* Nevele Country Club, Ellenville, NY, October 1984.

HULTH, A. (1982) Experimental osteoarthritis. *Acta Orthop. Scand.* **53**, 1–6.

JONES, R., SMITH E. and REISCH, J. (1978) Effects of medial meniscectomy in patients older than 40 years. *J. Bone Joint Surg.* **60**A, 783–786.

LUST, G. and WURSTER, N.B. (1987) On the pathogenesis of canine osteoarthritis. This volume.

MINNS, R.J. and MUCKLE, D.S. (1982) The role of the meniscus in an instability model of osteoarthritis in the rabbit knee. *Br. J. Exp. Pathol.* **63**, 18–24.

MOSKOWITZ, R. (1977) Experimentally induced joint lesions following partial meniscectomy in the rabbit. In: *Workshop on Models for Osteoarthritis.* University of Wales, Powys, Wales, 1977.

MUCKLE, D.S. (1982) Inflammatory involvement in osteoarthritis and lessons to be learnt from animal models. *Eur. J. Rheum. Inflamm.* **5**, 39–47.

O'BYRNE, E.M., QUINTAVALLA, J., STRAWINSKI, C., SCHRODER, H., BUTLER, M., COLOMBO, C., SWARTZENDRUBER, D. and STEINETZ, B. (1987) Towards therapy for the future: testing in cartilage–synovium co-cultures to detect potential cartilage-protective drugs. This volume.

O'BYRNE, E., STRAWINSKI, C., VASILENKO, P., QUINTAVALLA, J., ADELIZZI, R. and PHILLIPPS, M. (1984) Comparison of cartilage breakdown by human rheumatoid and osteoarthritic synovia when co-cultured in contact and at a distance. In: *Program of the 30th Annual Meeting of the Orthopaedic Research Society,* Atlanta, Georgia, February 1984, p. 312.

OXLUND, H., MANTHORPE, R. and VIIDIK, A. (1981) The biochemical properties of connective tissue in rabbits as influenced by short term treatment with glucocorticoid treatment. *J. Biomech.* **14**, 129–134.

PALMOSKI, M.J. and BRANDT, K.D. (1979) Effect of salicylate on proteoglycan metabolism in normal canine articular cartilage *in vitro. Arthritis Rheum.* **22**, 746–754.

PALMOSKI, M.J. and BRANDT, K.D. (1980) Effects of some non-steroidal anti-inflammatory drugs on proteoglycan metabolism and organisation in canine articular cartilage. *Arthritis Rheum.* **23**, 1010–1020.

PALMOSKI, M.J. and BRANDT, K.D. (1982a) Aspirin aggravates the degeneration of canine joint cartilage caused by immobilisation. *Arthritis Rheum.* **25**, 1333–1342.

PALMOSKI, M.J. and BRANDT, K.D. (1982b) Immobilisation of the knee prevents osteoarthritis after anterior cruciate ligament transection. *Arthritis Rheum.* **25**, 1201–1208.

PALMOSKI, M.J., COLYER, R.A. and BRANDT, K.D. (1980) Marked suppression by salicylate of the augmented proteoglycan synthesis in osteoarthritic cartilage. *Arthritis Rheum.* **23**, 83–91.

PANAGIDES, J., LANDES, M. and SLOBODA, A. (1980) Destruction of articular cartilage by arthritic synovium *in vitro*: Mechanism of breakdown and effect of indomethacin and prednisolone. *Agents Actions* **10**, 22–30.

ROSNER, I.A., GOLDBERG, V., GETZY, L. and MOSKOWITZ, R. (1979) Effects of estrogen on cartilage and experimentally induced arthritis. *Arthritis Rheum.* **22**, 52–58.

ROSNER, I.A., GOLDBERG, V., GETZY, L. and MOSKOWITZ, R.W. (1980) A trial of intra-articular orgotein, a superoxide dismutase, in experimentally-induced arthritis. *J. Rheumatol.* **7**, 24–29.

ROSNER, I.A., MALEMUD, C.J., GOLDBERG, V., PAPAY, R. and MOSKOWITZ, R.W. (1981) Tamoxifen therapy of experimental osteoarthritis. *Arthritis Rheum.* **24**, S69.

SABISTON, E. and ADAMS, M. (1985) Catabolin production by synovium from an experimental osteoarthritis. In: *Program of the 31st Annual Meeting of the Orthopaedic Research Society,* Las Vegas, Nevada, January 1985, p. 263.

SCHRODER, H., QUINTAVALLA, J., O'BYRNE, E. and STEINETZ, B. (1984) Synovial cathepsin B in a rabbit model of osteoarthritis. In: *Program of the 30th Annual Meeting of the Orthopaedic*

Research Society, Atlanta, Georgia, February 1984, p. 349.

SCHWARTZ, E. and GREENWALD, R. (1980) Experimental models of osteoarthritis. *Bull. Rheum. Dis.* **30**, 1030–1033.

STEINBERG, J., TSUKAMOTO, S. and SLEDGE, C. (1979) A tissue culture model of cartilage breakdown in rheumatoid arthritis. III. Effects of antirheumatic drugs. *Arthritis Rheum.* **22**, 877–885.

STEINETZ, B., BEACH, V. and ELDEN, H. (1966) Some effects of hormones on contractile properties of rat tail tendon collagen. *Endocrinology* **79**, 1047–1052.

STEINETZ, B.G., COLOMBO, C., BUTLER, M., O'BYRNE, E.M. and STEELE, R.E. (1981) Animal models of osteoarthritis: Possible applications in a drug development program. *Curr. Ther. Res.* **30**, S60–S75.

STEINETZ, B., COLOMBO, C., BUTLER, M., O'BYRNE, E. and SWARTZENDRUBER, D. (1984) Pathophysiological studies on a rabbit model of osteoarthritis. In: *Proceedings of the First World Conference on Inflammation*, Venice, Italy, April 1984, p. 20.

STEINETZ, B., SWARTZENDRUBER, D., COLOMBO, C., BUTLER, M., O'BYRNE, E., WURSTER, N. and LUST, G. (1985) New parameters for evaluation of disease severity in a rabbit model of osteoarthritis. In: *Proceedings of the Second International Conference of the Inflammation Research Association*, Nevele Country Club, Ellenville, NY, October 1984.

STEPHENS, R., GHOSH, P. and TAYLOR, T. (1979) The pathogenesis of osteoarthrosis. *Med. Hypotheses* **5**, 809–816.

SWARTZENDRUBER, D., COLOMBO, C., BUTLER, M., HICKMAN, L., WOODWORTH, M. and STEINETZ, B. (1987) Cellular changes in synovium and meniscus of a rabbit model of osteoarthritis induced by partial meniscectomy. This volume.

TELHAG, H. (1973) Effect of tranexamic acid (Cyclokapron[R]) on the synthesis of chondroitin sulfate and the content of hexosamine in the same fractions of normal and degenerated joint cartilage in the rabbit. *Acta Orthop. Scand.* **44**, 249–255.

TROYER, H. (1982) Experimental models of osteoarthritis: A review. *Semin. Arthritis Rheum.* **11**, 362–374.

WILHELMI, G. and FAUST, R. (1976) Suitability of the C57 black mouse as an experimental model for the study of skeletal changes due to ageing. With special reference to osteoarthrosis and its response to tribenoside. *Pharmacology* **14**, 289–296.

WOOD, D., IHRIE, E., DINARELLO, C. and COHEN, P. (1983) Isolation of an interleukin-1-like factor from human synovium joint effusions. *Arthritis Rheum.* **26**, 975–982.

Chapter 8

Bone Destruction in Osteoarthritis and the Possible Role of Anti-inflammatory Drugs

L. SOLOMON*

Department of Orthopaedic Surgery, University of the Witwatersrand, Johannesburg, South Africa

*Now at The Medical School, University of Bristol, and Southmead Hospital, Bristol, UK.

SUMMARY

Sometimes the articular destruction in osteoarthritis (OA) is unusually rapid and severe, an effect which has been attributed to administration of anti-inflammatory drugs. To test this hypothesis, radiological changes in the hip joint have been assessed in two age- and sex-matched groups of patients, one group receiving high doses of indomethacin (at least 100 mg/day) or indomethacin with other nonsteroidal anti-inflammatory drugs (NSAIDs) and analgesics for a year, and the other either ibuprofen or fenbufen in moderate doses or analgesics alone.

At the first examination the severity of radiographic changes was similar in the two groups, but at the end of one year 25% of joints in the indomethacin-treated group showed unequivocal loss of articular width or progressive bone destruction, compared with only 10% in the other group, a statistically significant difference. One indomethacin-treated patient showed rapid joint deterioration even within this short time.

There is no firm evidence that adequate analgesia *per se* predisposes to excessive bone destruction. There is an alternative explanation for the phenomenon: that certain NSAIDs affect cartilage and bone structure directly, but whether and under what conditions they do so by inhibiting glycosaminoglycan synthesis is not clear.

The term 'osteoarthritis' or 'osteoarthrosis' (OA) covers a number of clinical syndromes which may be subsets of a single pathological entity or entirely different disorders which share certain morphological features that appear in current definitions.

In a previous study of 150 patients with OA of the hip an attempt was made to separate the various pathogenetic types of disorder (Solomon and Schnitzler, 1983). This is necessary if one is to investigate the effect of anti-inflammatory therapy on the natural progression of the disease. Cases were classified according to the presence or absence of some local anatomical defect which could predispose to *mechanical overload*, and according to the presence or absence of some primary disorder which could cause *cartilage degeneration*. New bone formation and remodelling were also assessed: this reparative response was most marked in joints with anatomical abnormalities and least evident in those with previous inflammatory disease.

It is likely that the articular changes in OA are due to a combination of these factors, with certain features predominating in each particular case. Those showing well marked subchondral sclerosis and osteophyte formation were called 'hypertrophic OA' (Fig. 1), and those with minimal evidence of remodelling were called 'atrophic OA' (Fig. 2).

Among the latter group of patients were several (four out of 150) who developed unusually rapid and severe articular destruction (Fig. 3). This was attributed to the administration of certain nonsteroidal anti-inflammatory drugs — especially indomethacin in high dosage — and the cases were regarded as further examples of the drug-induced arthropathy previously described (Solomon, 1973). However, three of these patients had evidence of chondrocalcinosis and in two calcium pyrophosphate dihydrate (CPPD) crystals were subsequently demonstrated in the joint synovium.

These studies provided three possible explanations for the rapidly progressive bone destruction that sometimes occurs in OA of the hip: (a) it could be a severe form of the atrophic response that is inherent in certain types of OA from the outset; (b) it could be a form of crystal arthropathy similar to that described by McCarty (1976) and Dieppe *et al.* (1982); and (c) it might result from the administration of anti-inflammatory drugs.

In order to pursue the last of these possibilities, radiographic changes were assessed in patients receiving long-term anti-inflammatory therapy and in a control group of patients.

PATIENTS AND METHODS

Only patients with OA of the hip who did not require surgery and who were maintained on simple analgesics or nonsteroidal anti-inflammatory drugs (NSAIDs) for at least a year were considered for inclusion in this study. Among these patients two 'experimental' categories were defined: (a) those receiving

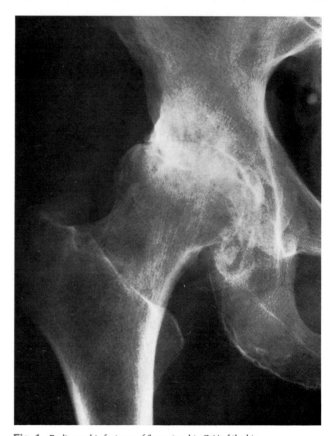

Fig. 1. Radiographic features of 'hypertrophic OA' of the hip.

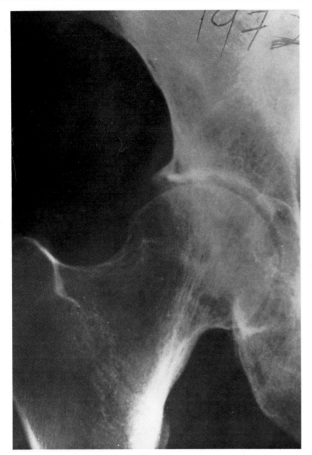

Fig. 2. Radiographic features of 'atrophic OA' of the hip.

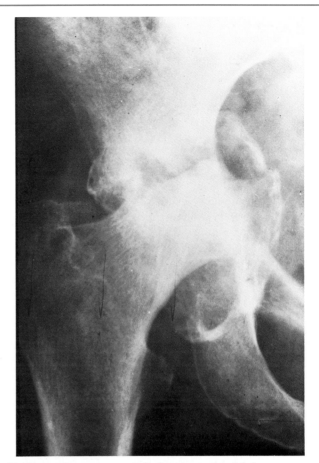

Fig. 3. Rapidly progressive articular destruction in OA of the hip.

indomethacin in large doses (minimum 100 mg per day) or indomethacin plus other NSAIDs and analgesics continuously for a year (20 patients, 27 hips); and (b) a similar group receiving either ibuprofen or fenbufen in moderate dosage, or analgesics such as paracetamol without any NSAID (31 patients, 41 hips). Age and sex distribution were comparable in the two groups (Table I).

Radiographs of the hips were obtained on admission to the Hip Clinic and at six-monthly intervals thereafter. Initial and one-year radiographs for all cases were assessed together without reference to the treatment category. The following signs of deterioration were noted: measurable thinning of the 'joint space', loss of subchondral bone, appearance of new cysts, and distortion of the femoral head. The object was to find the frequency, rather than the severity, of radiographic deterioration over the one-year period; no attempt was made to grade the changes.

RESULTS

The severity of radiographic changes at the first examination was similar in these two groups of patients.

Seven of the joints in the 'indomethacin group' (25%) and four in the 'control group' (10%) showed unequivocal loss of articular width or progressive bone destruction over the period of one year (Table II). This difference is statistically significant. One patient in the indomethacin group showed rapid progression even in this short period (Fig. 4).

DISCUSSION

In a review of 294 cases of coxarthrosis, Rønningen and Langeland (1979) found that progression of destructive changes

Table I. Age and sex distribution of patients with OA of the hips

	Number of patients	Number of hips	M:F	Median age (years)
Patients on indomethacin	20	27	7:13	61·2
Patients on other drugs	31	41	12:19	63·4

Table II. Proportion of patients showing progressive articular destruction over one year

	Number of hips	Number with articular destruction	Percentage
Patients on indomethacin	27	7	25
Patients on other drugs	41	4	10

occurred more frequently and that the severity of bone destruction was significantly greater in patients treated with indomethacin than in a control group; they concluded that the anti-inflammatory drug 'might have a deleterious effect' on joints

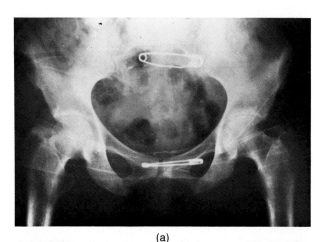

(a)

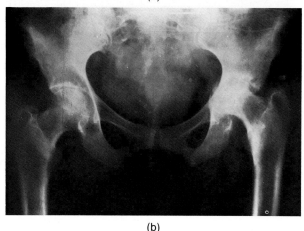

(b)

Fig. 4. Radiographs of the hips of a patient in the indomethacin group taken at an interval of 13 months.

already altered by osteoarthritis. The results of the present study support the primary observation that continuous treatment with indomethacin is associated with an increased frequency of cartilage and bone destruction in osteoarthritic hips. That this often occurs despite the subjective improvement in symptoms leads perhaps too easily to the conclusion that it results from the effective control of pain. There is as yet no firm evidence that adequate analgesia *per se* predisposes to excessive bone destruction; in almost all the reports on this phenomenon an anti-inflammatory drug has been implicated.

An alternative explanation is that certain NSAIDs may directly affect cartilage and bone structure. For a long time it has been known that anti-inflammatory drugs can inhibit glycosaminoglycan synthesis (Whitehouse and Bostrom, 1962), and the same action has been demonstrated *in vitro* in human cartilage obtained from femoral heads during operations (McKenzie *et al.*, 1976). Perhaps significantly, the latter authors found this effect in some specimens but not others; the precise conditions in which these changes are produced have yet to be defined.

REFERENCES

Dieppe, P.A., Alexander, G.J.M., Jones, H.E., Doherty, M., Scott, D.G.I., Manhire, A. and Watt, I. (1982) Pyrophosphate arthropathy: a clinical and radiological study of 105 cases. *Ann. Rheum. Dis.* **41**, 371–376.

McCarty, D.J. (1976) Calcium pyrophosphate dihydrate crystal deposition disease—1975. *Arthritis Rheum.* **19**, 275–285.

McKenzie, L.S., Horsburgh, B.A., Ghosh, P. and Taylor, T.K.F. (1976) Effect of anti-inflammatory drugs on sulphated glycosaminoglycan synthesis in aged human articular cartilage. *Ann. Rheum. Dis.* **35**, 487–497.

Rønningen, H. and Langeland, N. (1979) Indomethacin treatment in osteoarthritis of the hip joint. *Acta Orthop. Scand.* **50**, 169–174.

Solomon, L. (1973) Drug-induced arthropathy and necrosis of the femoral head. *J. Bone Joint Surg.* **55**B, 246–261.

Solomon, L. and Schnitzler, C.M. (1983) Pathogenetic types of coxarthrosis and implications for treatment. *Arch. Orthop. Traum. Surg.* **101**, 259–261.

Whitehouse, M.W. and Bostrom, H. (1962) The effect of some anti-inflammatory (anti-rheumatic) drugs on the metabolism of connective tissue. *Biochem. Pharmacol.* **11**, 1175–1201.

Chapter 9

Towards Therapy for the Future: Testing in Cartilage-synovium Co-cultures to Detect Potential Cartilage-protective Drugs

E. M. O'BYRNE, J. C. QUINTAVALLA, C. STRAWINSKI, H. SCHRODER, M. C. BUTLER, C. COLOMBO, D. SWARTZENDRUBER and B. G. STEINETZ

Research and Development Department, Pharmaceuticals Division, CIBA-GEIGY Corporation, Ardsley, New York, USA

SUMMARY

We report here our use of synovium-induced degradation of cartilage to measure the inhibitory activity of drugs which could prove useful in the treatment of osteoarthrosis. In this test system the proteoglycan matrix of bovine nasal septal cartilage is labelled *in vitro* by incorporation of sulphur-35 into glycosaminoglycan. The cartilage is then incubated with rabbit synovium explants for four days with each test drug, hydrolysed, and the cartilage hydrolysate counted. From the extent of ^{35}S release the percentage inhibition of matrix degradation in the presence of each drug, as against control, can be calculated.

Drugs inhibiting ^{35}S release in this system are then tested for inhibition of cartilage-degrading enzymes and of the response of living cartilage to catabolic factors in rabbit synovium-conditioned medium. Either component can be preincubated with drug before co-culture.

The model can also be used to study cartilage destruction produced by synovium of rabbits with surgically-induced osteoarthrosis.

INTRODUCTION

An *in vitro* cartilage-synovium co-culture bioassay has been applied at Ciba-Geigy to identify novel compounds that inhibit proteoglycan degradation in hyaline cartilage. Compounds preselected in this 'joint in a jar' assay subsequently undergo *in vivo* evaluation as potential therapeutic agents for degenerative joint disease.

For drug testing, ^{35}S-labelled bovine nasal cartilage is co-cultured *at a distance* from normal rabbit synovium in a *serum-free* medium. A co-culture model such as this can detect drugs that inhibit cartilage degradation by a variety of mechanisms, including: inhibition of production, secretion, and/or activation of degradative enzymes and/or synovial-mediating factors (catabolins); inhibition of chondrocyte response to catabolins; and direct inhibition of enzymatic activities.

BACKGROUND

Fell and Jubb (1977) were the first to compare changes in cartilage matrix components during incubation of living cartilage in contact with synovium with those observed when the same tissue types were cultured at a distance from each other in the same medium. Dead cartilage was used as one type of control. Living cartilage in contact with synovium lost both proteoglycan and collagen; dead cartilage lost proteoglycan but less collagen. Proteoglycan was also lost when living cartilage was incubated at a distance from synovium but in the same culture medium; however, dead cartilage was not degraded under these conditions. These observations led to the hypothesis that the synovium exerts two distinct effects: a direct enzymatic action on cartilage matrix and an indirect effect mediated through the living chondrocytes.

In vitro studies of mechanisms by which synovium and other cells and tissues modify cartilage proteoglycan matrix metabolism have employed a variety of co-culture systems (Steinberg *et al.*, 1979a; Crossley and Hunneyball, 1982, for review). Co-cultures containing human rheumatoid synovium in contact with bovine nasal cartilage (Steinberg *et al.*, 1979c) and traumatised normal pig synovium in contact with pig articular cartilage (Crossley and Hunneyball, 1982) have been used to monitor effects of antirheumatic drugs on cartilage matrix depletion. Dingle and Saklatvala (Dingle, 1979; Dingle, 1981; Saklatvala, 1981; Saklatvala and Dingle, 1981) have focused on identification of factors released by the synovium into the medium which are capable of mediating cartilage degradation. The factor(s) responsible for stimulation of chondrocyte-mediated destruction of the proteoglycan matrix was dubbed 'catabolin'. Factors that induce cartilage degradation are also produced by mononuclear cells (Jasin and Dingle, 1981), macrophages (Deshmukh-Phadke *et al.*, 1978; 1980; Ridge *et al.*, 1980) and vascular tissue (Jubb, 1982; Deker and Dingle, 1982).

METHODS

'Joint in a jar' screen

Bovine nasal septum cartilage is dissected into 300–400 roughly equivalent explants measuring about $1 \times 1 \times 2$ mm (O'Byrne *et al.*, 1983a). The proteoglycan matrix is labelled during incubation in 50 ml sulphate-free Joklik's modification of Dulbecco's Minimum Essential Medium to which has been added 8 mCi Na$_2$^{35}SO$_4$ (Dingle *et al.*, 1977). Synovial tissue is obtained from normal male rabbits by removing the infrapatellar fat pad and its synovial lining and cutting it into eight pie-shaped explants. Washed ^{35}S-labelled cartilage slices are co-cultured with synovial explants in 1·0 ml Dulbecco's Minimal Essential Medium containing 0·5% Bacto-peptone, 25 mM HEPES, 100 units/ml penicillin, 100 μg/ml streptomycin and 2·5 μ/ml fungizone. Because the rabbit synovial lining is attached to the infrapatellar fat pad it floats, creating a natural separation from the cartilage at the bottom of the culture dish (Fig. 1). After four days' incubation, radioactivity is determined in an aliquot of culture medium and in the sample of the remaining cartilage following hydrolysis to permit calculation of the percentage of ^{35}S released into the medium.

To compare the degrees to which proteoglycan matrix components and collagen fragments were released into the medium during a five-day incubation, hydroxyproline in aliquots of culture media and cartilage hydrolysate from four cartilage explants cultured alone and four cartilage-synovium co-cultures

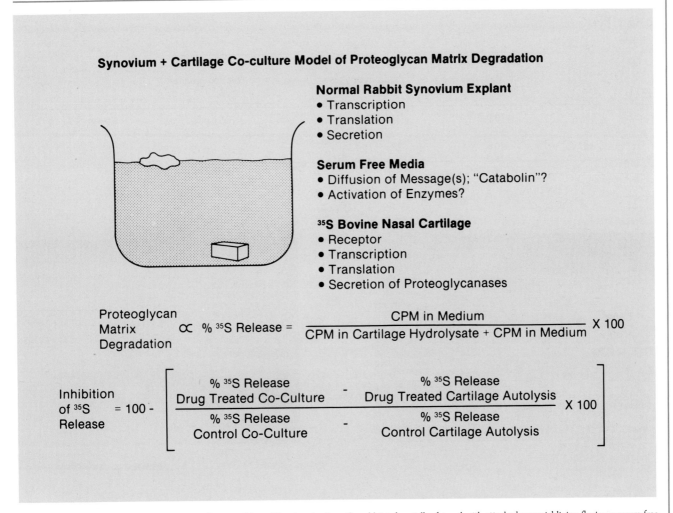

Fig. 1. Diagram of synovium + cartilage co-culture model used for drug testing; the rabbit infrapatellar fat pad with attached synovial lining floats on serum-free medium at a distance from ^{35}S-labelled bovine nasal hyaline cartilage. (CPM = cartilage proteoglycan matrix.)

was determined by the method of Woessner (1961). In contrast to the marked stimulation of ^{35}S release in co-cultures, the hydroxyproline released into the co-culture medium was not greater than that observed with cartilage cultured alone (Table I).

Latent neutral metallo-proteoglycanase and latent collagenase activity are present in both synovium-conditioned medium and cartilage-plus-synovium co-culture medium. Crossley and Hunneyball (1982) noted that for pig synovial collagenase to degrade collagen in pig articular cartilage it was essential that the two tissues were in contact.

Pattern of matrix depletion: histochemistry and autoradiography

Slices of ^{35}S-labelled bovine nasal cartilage were fixed in 10% formalin containing 1% sodium acetate and 7% disodium EDTA,

dehydrated in alcohol, cleared in xylene, and embedded in paraffin. For autoradiographic analysis (O'Byrne et al., 1983b), 6 μm sections were affixed to glass slides, deparaffinised and hydrated. Slides were dipped in NTB2 Kodak Nuclear Track Emulsion, dried and exposed 24 hours in light-tight slide boxes. Sections were developed in Kodak D19 Developer and fixed in Kodak Acid Fixer. The cartilage sections were then stained with safranin 0 for sulphated proteoglycans and counterstained with Fast Green FCF.

At the start of the incubation period, stained microscopic autoradiographs of ^{35}S-labelled bovine nasal cartilage show an even distribution of safranin 0 staining throughout the matrix, with more intense staining in the pericellular region of the chondrocyte lacunae. The ^{35}S incorporated into newly synthesised proteoglycan is indicated by silver grains in the pericellular region of chondrocytes throughout the tissue. In the cartilage cultured alone (Fig. 2c, left) there was a slight uniform depletion

Table I. Differential degradation of proteoglycan and collagen in cartilage explants and cartilage co-cultured with synovium at a distance after five days' incubation

	Culture medium hydroxyproline (µg)	Cartilage hydrolysate hydroxyproline (µg)	% Hydroxyproline release	% ³⁵S release
Cartilage	< 10·0	312 ± 31·9	< 3·2 ± 0·3	34·6 ± 3·9
Cartilage + synovium co-culture	< 10·0	285 ± 13·0	< 3·5 ± 0·15	74·0 ± 13·4

Day 4

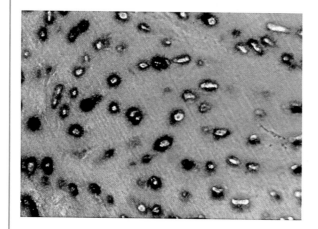 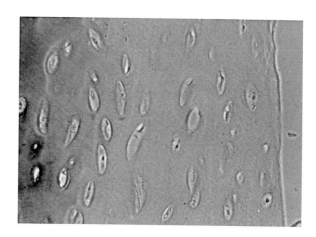

Day 6

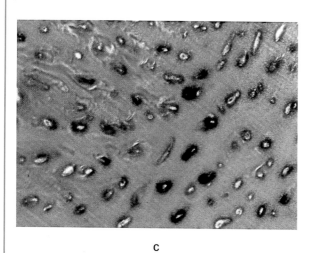 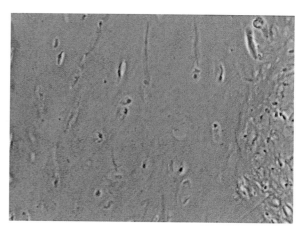

c   c + s

Fig. 2. Safranin 0-stained ³⁵S-labelled phase microautoradiographs of bovine nasal cartilage. *Top*, Day 4: Cartilage autolysis (c, left). Safraninophilia is uniform with dense silver grains around chondrocytes. Cartilage co-cultured with synovium (c + s, right). There is a loss of safraninophilia and a decreased ³⁵S reduction of silver. The depletion of the proteoglycan matrix has proceeded from the external surfaces of the cartilage toward the centre of the slices. *Bottom*, Day 6: Cartilage cultured alone (c, left). Both safraninophilia and ³⁵S are still evident. Cartilage co-cultured with synovium (c + s, right). Depletion of both safraninophilia and ³⁵S has progressed from the surface inward.

of staining and silver grains indicative of radiosulphate after four (top) and six (bottom) days' incubation. In cartilage-plus-synovium co-cultures there was a progressive loss of safranin 0 staining and radioactivity from the surface of the explants (Fig. 2, c + s, left). Autoradiographs of co-cultured cartilage indicate pericellular accumulation of ^{35}S in inner regions of cartilage that stained with safranin 0 while peripheral areas negative for safranin 0 also lacked pericellular ^{35}S. These static observations do not reveal evidence for local degradation of matrix in the micro-environments of stimulated chondrocytes (Dingle and Dingle, 1980). However, the release of ^{35}S into the medium was not stimulated when live synovium was co-cultured with killed cartilage, indicating an essential active role of living chondrocytes in proteoglycan degradation.

ACTIVITY OF ANTIRHEUMATIC DRUGS

Glucocorticoids in concentrations of 10^{-6} M afforded up to 50% inhibition of matrix depletion in our co-culture model. These observations are in agreement with the matrix-protective activity of glucocorticoids in co-cultures of bovine nasal cartilage in contact with human rheumatoid synovium (Steinberg *et al.*, 1979b; 1979c). Indomethacin was inactive at 10^{-4} M in this model, which is in agreement with data from other co-culture systems (Crossley and Hunneyball, 1982; Steinberg *et al.*, 1979c). Penicillamine had no cartilage-protective properties in this or other co-culture models (Crossley and Hunneyball, 1982; Jacoby, 1980). Tamoxifen, which prevented cartilage destruction in a rabbit model of OA (Rosner *et al.*, 1981), was active at 1×10^{-4} M but not at 1×10^{-5} M in co-culture.

FUTURE THERAPEUTIC INTERVENTION: INHIBITION OF CARTILAGE DEGENERATION

Dr Helen Muir (1977) has pointedly stated: 'The drugs that are at present prescribed for osteoarthrosis have been developed for the treatment of entirely different diseases. Whether they are of real benefit to patients is quite questionable and some

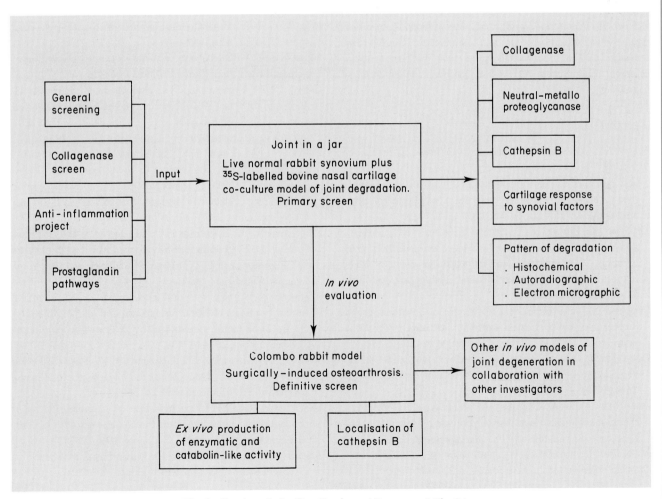

Fig. 3. Chondroprotective Drug Development Programme at Ciba-Geigy.

109

may even be harmful particularly if given for long periods of time. To develop drugs specifically for osteoarthrosis therefore presents a challenge to the pharmaceutical industry, but the thinking that has gone into the development of antirheumatic drugs should be discarded.' For therapeutic intervention in human OA to be feasible, one must postulate that the disease is metabolic, not simply a matter of wear and tear on the joints. There is a growing body of evidence from human and animal studies that support this possibility. Indeed, two different laboratories have reported significant chondroprotective effects of drugs in surgically-induced OA in rabbits (Rosner *et al.*, 1981; Colombo *et al.*, 1983; Butler *et al.*, 1983). Our laboratory is currently investigating the possible role of synovial factors (both enzymatic and catabolin-like) in surgically induced OA and attempting to correlate these findings with those obtained using our co-culture system.

At Ciba-Geigy our drug-testing programme (Fig. 3) is based on inhibition of cartilage degradation in organ culture followed by *in vivo* evaluation in surgically induced OA in rabbits, to discover chondroprotective agents for degenerative joint diseases.

Since this manuscript was first submitted a second-generation organ culture screen based on degradation of live bovine nasal cartilage by an operationally-pure, enzyme-free synovial catabolin (Quintavalla *et al.*, 1984) has been implemented at Ciba-Geigy.

REFERENCES

BUTLER, M., COLOMBO, C., HICKMAN, L., O'BYRNE, E., STEELE, R., STEINETZ, B., QUINTAVALLA, J. and YOKOYAMA, N. (1983) A new model of osteoarthritis in rabbits: III. Evaluation of anti-osteoarthritic effects of selected drugs administered intra-articularly. *Arthritis Rheum.* **26**, 1380–1386.

COLOMBO, C., BUTLER, M., HICKMAN, L., SELWYN, M., CHART, J. and STEINETZ, B. (1983) A new model of osteoarthritis (OA) in rabbits: II. Evaluation of anti-osteoarthritic effects of selected antirheumatic drugs administered systemically. *Arthritis Rheum.* **26**, 1132–1139.

CROSSLEY, M.J. and HUNNEYBALL, I.M. (1982) Biochemical and pharmacological studies on synovium-cartilage interactions in organ culture. *Eur. J. Rheum. Inflamm.* **5**, 15–29.

DEKER, R.S. and DINGLE, J.T. (1982) Cardiac catabolic factor: the degradation of the heart valve intercellular matrix. *Sciences* **215**, 987–989.

DESHMUKH-PHADKE, K., LAWRENCE, M. and NANDA, S. (1978) Synthesis of collagenase and neutral protease by articular chondrocytes: Stimulation by a macrophage-derived factor. *Biochem. Biophys. Res. Commun.* **85**, 490–496.

DESHMUKH-PHADKE, K., NANDA, S. and LEE, K. (1980) Macrophage factors that induce neutral protease secretion by normal rabbit chondrocytes. *Eur. J. Biochem.* **104**, 175–180.

DINGLE, J.T. (1979) Recent studies on the control of joint damage: the contributions of the Strangeways Research Laboratory. *Ann. Rheum. Dis.* **38**, 201–214.

DINGLE, J.T. (1981) Catabolin-A cartilage catabolic factor from synovium. *Clin. Orthop.* **156**, 219–231.

DINGLE, J.T., BLOW, A.M., BARRETT, A.J. and MARTIN, P.E.N. (1977) Proteoglycan degrading enzymes: a radiochemical method and the detection of a new enzyme cathepsin F. *Biochem. J.* **167**, 775–785.

DINGLE, J.T. and DINGLE, T.T. (1980) The site of cartilage matrix degradation. *Biochem. J.* **190**, 431–438.

FELL, H.B. and JUBB, R.W. (1977) The effect of synovial tissue on the breakdown of articular cartilage in organ culture. *Arthritis Rheum.* **20**, 1359–1371.

JACOBY, R.K. (1980) Effect of homologous synovial membrane on adult human articular cartilage in organ culture and failure to influence it with D-penicillamine. *Ann. Rheum. Dis.* **39**, 53–58.

JASIN, H.E. and DINGLE, J.T. (1981) Human mononuclear cell factors mediate matrix degradation through chondrocyte activation. *Arthritis Rheum.* **24**, 106S.

JUBB, R.W. (1982) Breakdown of articular cartilage by vascular tissue. *J. Pathol.* **136**, 333–343.

MUIR, H. (1977) Molecular approaches to the understanding of osteoarthrosis. *Ann. Rheum. Dis.* **36**, 199–208.

O'BYRNE, E.M., QUINTAVALLA, J.C., STRAWINSKI, C., SCHRODER, H. and STEINETZ, B.G. (1983a) Normal synovial tissue co-cultured with ^{35}S-labeled cartilage as an *in vitro* model of degenerative joint disease. *Trans. 29th Ann. Orthop. Res. Soc.*, p. 398.

O'BYRNE, E.M., BUTLER, M.C., SCHRODER, H.C., QUINTAVALLA, J.C., HICKMAN, L.Y., STRAWINSKI, C., SWARTZENDRUBER, D. and STEINETZ, B.G. (1983b) Histochemical and autoradiographic analysis of ^{35}S-labeled cartilage co-cultured with normal synovium. *Trans. 29th Ann. Orthop. Res. Soc.*, p. 322.

QUINTAVALLA, J.C., SCHRODER, H.C., PHILLIPS, M.A. and O'BYRNE, E.M. (1984) Degradation of bovine nasal cartilage by factors secreted by bovine synovium in culture. *2nd Int. Conf. Inflamm. Res. Assoc.*

RIDGE, S.C., ORONSKY, A.L. and KERWAR, S.S. (1980) Induction of the synthesis of latent collagenase and latent proteoglycanase by a factor synthesised by activated macrophages. *Arthritis Rheum.* **23**, 448–454.

ROSNER, I.A., MALEMUD, C.J., GOLDBERG, V.M., PAPAY, R.S. and MOSKOWITZ, R.W. (1981) Tamoxifen therapy of experimental osteoarthritis. *Arthritis Rheum.* **24**, S69.

SAKLATVALA, J. (1981) Characterisation of catabolin, the major product of pig synovium tissue that induces resorption of cartilage proteoglycan *in vitro*. *Biochem. J.* **199**, 705–714.

SAKLATVALA, J. and DINGLE, J.T. (1981) Identification of catabolin, a protein from synovium which induces degradation of cartilage in organ culture. *Biochem. Biophys. Res. Commun.* **96**, 1225–1231.

STEINBERG, J., SLEDGE, C., NOBLE, J. and STIRRAT, C. (1979a) A tissue culture model of cartilage breakdown in rheumatoid arthritis — quantitative aspects of proteoglycan release. *Biochem. J.* **180**, 403–412.

STEINBERG, J., TSUKAMOTO, S. and SLEDGE, C.B. (1979b) Hydrocortisone inhibition of cartilage breakdown in rheumatoid arthritis—an *in vitro* model. *Trans. 25th Ann. Orthop. Res. Soc.*, p. 51.

STEINBERG, J., TSUKAMOTO, S. and SLEDGE, C. (1979c) A tissue culture model of cartilage degradation in rheumatoid arthritis. III. Effects of antirheumatic drugs. *Arthritis Rheum.* **22**, 877–885.

WOESSNER, J.F. (1961) The determination of hydroxyproline in tissue and protein samples containing small proportions of this amino acid. *Arch. Biochem. Biophys.* **93**, 440–447.

Chapter 10

Pharmacological Control of Osteoarthritis: A Realisable Goal?

MALCOLM I. V. JAYSON

Rheumatic Diseases Centre, Hope Hospital, University of Manchester, UK

INTRODUCTION

In order to suggest forms of treatment that will control osteoarthritis (OA) in a fundamental fashion it is necessary to consider the pathogenesis of this disorder. Two fundamental mechanisms are proposed as responsible for development of OA. In both, articular cartilage is stressed: either by an absolute excess load, or by a relative excess due to diminished cartilage resistance. The excessive resultant strain may cause collagen-fibre failure with resultant proteoglycan loss and cartilage softening. Alternatively stress causes release of degradative enzymes perhaps mediated via catabolin. These enzymes lead to proteoglycan degradation and loss. Cartilage softening in turn leads to a further increase in the relative strain with any load so that a vicious circle of collagen degradation develops. Repair phenomena including fibrosis of the joint capsule and osteophytosis occur and eventually the complex syndrome of OA develops.

Within these pathogenetic pathways are several possible points at which therapeutic intervention may have a fundamental effect on the development of OA. Although there has been a certain amount of experimental success so far, there is no good evidence that pharmacological control of OA has been achieved in man. I wish here to review the various types of approach and indicate directions that may be of interest for future studies. To my mind the priority at the present time is to identify the mechanisms underlying such intervention and to illustrate their potential for benefit. Initial work can be undertaken in animals to establish the principles involved. Once we have a clear idea of the fundamental mechanisms that should be influenced and the types of treatment that possess the desired properties, then we can proceed to the details of how to apply such principles in man.

OBJECTIVES OF TREATMENT

Pain relief

Analgesia can be achieved by drugs or by some of the physical methods of pain control which are in general use in pain clinics. It is clear that analgesia alone will not have a fundamental effect on OA; however, it is known that disuse may lead to cartilage fibril formation and, at the other extreme, excessive use may potentiate articular cartilage damage. It is possible that in animal models the progression of OA may be accelerated or prevented in relation to increased physical activity resulting from the analgesic actions of these compounds.

Control of inflammation

An element of secondary inflammation is common in OA, but its cause is not clear. It may be due to the production by detritus of mechanical or inflammatory changes, or calcium pyrophosphate or hydroxyapatite crystals.

Examination of synovial biopsy specimens may reveal chronic inflammatory-cell infiltration and sometimes it is difficult to distinguish synovial biopsy samples from those of patients with inflammatory arthritis. Some patients show an element of morning stiffness and may suffer transient inflammatory episodes within their joints.

There is no doubt that for most patients anti-inflammatory drugs provide better symptomatic relief than simple analgesics. Indeed there is some evidence that steroids, which have considerable anti-inflammatory potency but no analgesic action, provide considerable relief to some osteoarthritic patients when given by local injection and even on occasion when given by mouth. This is not a therapeutic recommendation but simply an important point in considering fundamental treatment mechanisms.

It is not clear, however, whether anti-inflammatory therapy has any effect on the course of OA. There are theoretical reasons for believing that it may even exacerbate joint damage. Professor Solomon provided some evidence that this occurs with indomethacin but such studies are always open to the criticism that the worst cases are the most likely to progress and to receive the most potent agents. This issue is still in considerable doubt.

Prevention of collagen-fibre damage

Relative or absolute overuse of the joints leads to failure of collagen fibres and the initiation of the osteoarthritic process. Careful consideration of the anatomical and biomechanical factors in each individual case helps in planning the surgical approach to treatment. A carefully planned osteotomy will shift the concentration of forces away from the area of damage and spread the load over a wider area. It may use the osteophyte as a load-bearing surface. Careful studies using serial radiographs have demonstrated the potential of articular cartilage for regrowth under such circumstances. The exciting observations to emerge from these studies are not only the results of specific forms of treatment but also that damaged cartilage has an inherent potential for recovery: the statement that cartilage once damaged has no powers to regenerate is incorrect. Under normal circumstances the stress causing cartilage damage continues so that no opportunity for repair arises. If the cartilage can be protected then it can regenerate like many other tissues.

Collagen damage may also be mediated by release of specific enzymes, in particular collagenases. These are found in synovial fluid, inflamed synovium and articular cartilage. Inhibitors of collagenase may occur naturally or perhaps be administered as therapy. It may be possible to prevent collagen-fibre damage by interfering with the formation or release of collagenases, by stimulating inhibitors or by administering them.

Enhancement of proteoglycan content

There are a number of potential mechanisms for increasing the proteoglycan content of articular cartilage. They may be considered as follows.

Synthesis

Human growth hormone when administered to animals increases proteoglycan synthesis and in particular cartilage synthesis. It has no direct effect on articular cartilage *in vitro* but its actions seem to be mediated via somatomedin, a product liberated when human growth hormone is incubated together with liver. In the future it may be possible to use somatomedin as a therapeutic compound for OA. Connective-tissue stimulating factor and connective-tissue activation peptide are liberated in chronic inflammation: they possess certain properties which seem desirable including promotion of proteoglycan synthesis. It may prove possible to use these compounds therapeutically.

Content

Supplementary proteoglycan has been given for the treatment of OA. The preparations include sulphated glycosaminoglycan, uridine diphosphate and cartilage/bone-marrow extract. Experimental work in animal models strongly suggests that they can prevent the development of OA, but despite extensive studies their value in human disease remains in doubt, partly due to the lack of adequate controls in clinical trials. The limited studies that have been conducted suggest some benefit but their results fail to achieve statistical significance. One major study was conducted on patients awaiting hip replacement who therefore had very severe advanced OA. They had probably reached a stage of severe cartilage damage by which time it is unlikely that any form of treatment could restore cartilage function.

Degradation

Proteoglycan is degraded by various enzymes, release of which may be inhibited by non-steroidal anti-inflammatory drugs or by steroids. Experimental studies have shown that these compounds are capable of inhibiting OA in experimental models of the disease and it may be that they have a potential for benefit in human OA. Detailed controlled studies will be required before this can be confirmed.

Numerous enzymes may be responsible for articular cartilage proteoglycan degradation. There are many inhibitors of these enzymes and it may be possible to employ them as therapeutic agents. It will however be difficult to identify which specific enzymes should be inhibited and to find a means of delivering the appropriate inhibitory substances into the cartilage, in particular to the pericellular environment where the enzymes are concentrated.

Catabolin release is inhibited by corticosteroids: perhaps steroids can prevent the progression of cartilage degradation. Alternatively, if catabolin turns out to be a specific molecule it may be possible to neutralise its effect by means of monoclonal antibodies or specific inhibitors.

Enhancements of repair phenomena

Much of the clinical problem of osteoarthritis is caused not by the articular cartilage damage but by the secondary repair phenomena. These include the development of osteophytes around the margin of the joint and fibrosis of the joint capsule. Corticosteroids given either systemically or by intra-articular or periarticular injection in animal models will interfere with these repair phenomena. Although at first sight this may not seem an appropriate form of treatment nevertheless it may provide the symptomatic relief that is required.

Enhancement of lubrication

Artificial lubricants have been injected into joints in an effort to improve joint mobility. Their use has not been successful. This may be because the stiffness of osteoarthritic joints arises primarily from the soft tissue surrounding the joint rather than being due to friction at the articular surfaces.

CONSTRAINTS ON THE STUDY OF TREATMENT OF OSTEOARTHRITIS

The long-term and slow evolution of osteoarthritis will place constraints on any treatment programme. It will be necessary to be able to predict the natural history of the disease and in particular to identify the patient likely to develop joint failure. In these patients it should be possible to provide forms of treatment and examine whether or not progress of osteoarthritis can be prevented or even reversed. The protracted nature of the disease dictates that treatment will be required in the long term and therefore must be given orally and be non-toxic. Important ethical considerations arise in such forms of treatment, and in undertaking clinical trials it will be necessary to demonstrate that the treatment is both effective and safe. In addition, to be effective, drugs must be well absorbed and reach adequate levels within the articular cartilage.

HOW DO WE ASSESS PROGRESSION OF OA?

In undertaking trials of long-term management of OA it is important to separate clearly the various components of the disease, which are as follows:

1. The inflammatory element
2. Articular cartilage damage
3. Bone damage
4. Repair phenomena, such as capsular fibrosis of osteoporosis.

Each of these reflects different aspects of OA and it is uncertain which is the most important with respect to clinical progression of the disease. As examples, there may be clear evidence of cartilage damage with gross radiological changes and no symptoms, or vice versa. Careful documentation of the various components of the clinical problem of OA will help elucidate the true requirements for successful treatment.

NUMBERS OF PATIENTS REQUIRED FOR CONTROLLED STUDIES

It is helpful to make an analysis of the probable numbers of patients required in order to be able to demonstrate statistically the benefits which may follow treatment. As an example it has been calculated that five years after meniscectomy the radiological prevalence of OA is 27%. If some form of treatment is successful it may reduce the prevalence to 15%. How many patients would be required to demonstrate this with a statistical significance of $P < 0.05$? Because of the long-term nature of the study we should assume that there will be poor compliance and the drop-out rate may well be as high as 40%. Using a power test of 80% we would need 464 patients to achieve the desired results and, with a power test of 95%, 830 patients would be required. These numbers are enormous and make controlled studies a formidable undertaking. Nevertheless careful consideration must be given to such studies if the management of the disease is to be improved.

HOW CAN PROGRESSION OF OA BE MEASURED IN MAN?

HOW CAN PROGRESSION OF OA BE MEASURED IN MAN?

There are at present no techniques for objective measurement of any of the pathological changes in a joint affected by OA. Neither the progression of the disease nor its response to treatment can be assessed quantitatively. Evaluation of individual patients therefore continues to rest mainly on qualitative criteria, based on clinical findings supported by special investigations, as outlined in the following contributions. At present, the lack of objective measures prevents accurate comparisons, both over time and between patients, thus hindering study of the natural history of OA and the conduct of clinical trials. Isotope methods may offer the best prospect for overcoming these limitations in the future.

Chapter 11

Clinical Assessment

E. C. HUSKISSON
St Bartholomew's Hospital, London, UK

If drugs were available which cured osteoarthritis (OA), measurement would be unnecessary. However, there is no prospect of a cure: current treatments probably do no more than relieve symptoms. The next step may be a disease-modifying drug the actions of which will resemble those of penicillamine in rheumatoid arthritis. It would be gratifying to be able to anticipate this development by devising appropriate measurements, and to know whether currently available treatments make the disease better in the long term, or perhaps worse. However, in other diseases, measurements seem to have been developed in response to available treatment, after the event rather than before it. The lack of measurements of outcome in OA may be taken as an indication of the lack of treatment to modify it, but the symptoms of the disease can certainly be measured and modified.

Little is known about the natural history of OA, but it is known to be slowly progressive in most cases, with long intervals between involvement of new joint sites, and any particular joint taking years to reach to the stage of failure. In a few cases OA is also known to be rapidly progressive. The time has come to document such anecdotal evidence and to record exactly what happens to different patients' joints over the years while their disease runs its course.

WHAT CAN BE MEASURED?

Available and useful variables for measurement in OA include pain, stiffness, joint tenderness and function, all of which are responsive to current treatment. Pain can be measured by means of simple descriptive and visual analogue scales. The severity of pain in OA and its response to non-steroidal anti-inflammatory drugs is very similar to that in rheumatoid arthritis. The duration of stiffness in the morning and after sitting can be measured, reflecting the degree of inflammation, of which these are characteristic symptoms. Tender joints can be counted and their severity or assessed by means of an articular index.

Function can be measured in a variety of ways, using descriptive or visual analogue scales, questionnaires or tests, such as walking time. There are two major problems and limitations, however: first, function is affected by many other factors including age, other diseases and motivation; and second, disability in OA is individual and variable. One patient may have severely affected hands and be unable to write, while another may have severely affected knees and be unable to walk. One does not work, while the other cannot. Even when two patients have similar disease in the same joint, they may have quite different problems because their lifestyle is different. It is nevertheless important to assess function and thus to develop accurate methods of measurement.

Swelling is difficult to measure. Although the number of swollen joints can readily be counted, no satisfactory method has been developed to show treatment changes in a single joint such as the knee. Osteoarthritic joints are warm and show increased isotopic uptake but these techniques have not yet been used to assess treatment effects.

WHAT SHOULD BE MEASURED?

Outcome should be measured. Patients with OA eventually need joint replacements, walking sticks, drugs, social security and the help of others. They have more and more involved joints as time goes on, and the state of those joints deteriorates, but these factors are not easy to measure. However, individual patients can be counted, and there is a need to know what proportion of a large number of patients with OA will need hip or knee replacement. A large number of patients will need to be studied because it is known that most will not require an operation. It would be convenient if some common measure such as money could be found in which to express and compare their disparate outcomes. It would be unlikely to be widely acceptable, however, since it would fail to impress the clinician or the patient, who would wish to see tangible benefits such as pain relief and independence: neither would they be impressed by the 'Osteoarthritis Economic Outcome Indicator'.

X-ray changes may be a useful guide to disease progression, as they have been in rheumatoid arthritis. There is certainly a need for methods of assessing the radiological changes of OA and documenting their progression. It will also be important to show how radiological deterioration is related to clinical status.

Advances in the understanding of the disease process may also provide new measurements. In particular, biochemical changes in cartilage may become measurable, and may reflect disease activity and progression, but they will not replace clinical measurements such as pain. We shall always need to know whether the patient actually feels better, as well as showing that the disease process is controlled.

WHAT MEASURES TO CHOOSE?

The choice of measurements in a particular study will always depend on the aims of that study. One designed to show that a particular treatment relieves symptoms must measure symptoms. One designed to investigate the possibility that treatment alters the outcome of the disease must measure the outcome in terms which are of established relevance to both patient and physician. Such a study may also include measurement of symptoms since we shall always want to be sure that patients *feel* better as well as *being* better. Improved radiological and biochemical measures of the disease process offer the possibility of useful supporting evidence.

SELECT BIBLIOGRAPHY

DOYLE, D.V., DIEPPE, P.A., SCOTT, J. and HUSKISSON, E.C. (1981) An articular index for the assessment of osteoarthritis. *Ann. Rheum. Dis.* **40**, 75–78.

HUSKISSON, E.C. (1974) Measurements of pain. *Lancet* **ii**, 1127–1131.

HUSKISSON, E.C. (1979) Osteoarthritis: changing concepts in pathogenesis and treatment. *Postgrad. Med.* **65**, 97–108.

Proceedings of the conference on outcome measures in rheumatological clinical trials (1982) *J. Rheumatol.* **9**, 753–806.

SCOTT, P.J. and HUSKISSON, E.C. (1977) Measurements of functional capacity with visual analogue scales. *Rheum. Rehab.* **16**, 257–259.

Chapter 12

Arthroscopy in the Assessment of the Progress of Osteoarthritis

J. NOBLE

University of Manchester, UK

A radiologist, an orthopaedic surgeon, or a pathologist may take very different views of OA, and its pathological or radiological features are certainly much commoner than symptoms which might be conventionally ascribed to them. Four decades ago in a classical monograph on the necropsy incidence of joint disease Bennet et al. (1942) observed that the 'articulations remain normal for a short time following complete maturation'. In a recent study Fahmy et al. (1981) found evidence of articular degeneration in 98% of the 115 knees which they examined at necropsy. In 1912 Beitzke was probably the first to indicate the frequency of 'OA' in the general population from necropsy studies. In his work 60% of those under 40 years old and 95% over that age showed naked-eye features of OA. In a study of meniscal degeneration, closely allied to OA, Noble and Hamblen (1975) found at least one horizontal cleavage lesion in 60 of their 100 necropsy subjects. In a subsequent study Noble (1976) could only elicit typical symptoms of such a lesion in 5% of a similar, but living, geriatric population.

The problems which these observations pose in establishing a prospective study of methods to control or prevent the development of OA will be discussed below.

THE ARTHROSCOPE

The arthroscope is essentially a viewing light telescope which can be introduced through a cannula into a joint, such as the knee, to study in close and accurate detail the intra-articular structures and surfaces. Most arthroscopists will observe directly down the telescope, although it is possible to attach a television camera to the arthroscope and observe on a TV screen (Dandy, 1981). It is also possible to operate inside the joint using special instruments introduced through very small stab incisions in the skin. The operative edges of these instruments function within the joint, operated by the surgeon outside that joint. By these means operations such as synovial biopsy, meniscectomy, shaving of patella or removal of loose bodies may be accomplished. Such practice is commonplace in North America and to a lesser extent Northern Europe and Japan, where the technique was developed 60 years ago.

Meanwhile in Britain, in 1980, a leading authority on the knee has stated 'that arthroscopy has the most appeal for the least knowledgeable' (Smillie, 1980). Such reactions are not supportable when the evidence is examined. As a diagnostic procedure 25% of the menisci which, before the advent of arthroscopy, would have been removed are spared (De Haven and Collins, 1975; Dandy and Jackson, 1975; Noble and Erat, 1980). Arthroscopic meniscectomy can now be effected as a day procedure, whereas inpatient time for that operation by conventional surgical means in 1977 was $8\frac{1}{2}$ days in England and Wales (Noble et al., 1984).

Nevertheless the views which Smillie (1980) has enshrined remain popular, as the procedure is technically demanding, can

be time-consuming and ultimately has to be self-taught. The view that it should only be used in 'selected cases' reveals an ignorance of the difficulties in diagnosing intra-articular lesions, as shown by the clinical inaccuracy of doing so (Noble and Erat, 1980; Ireland et al., 1980), and also evades the essential point that the arthroscope, like the flute, is an instrument which, to be played well, requires regular practice.

HOW TO ASSESS ARTICULAR LESIONS

In the hands of an experienced arthroscopist the site, shape, extent and depth of lesions of the articular surface can be assessed. Such observations can be recorded on prepared graphic charts of the articular surfaces of the knee (analogous to a Mercator map projection). This, in turn, can be augmented quite easily by taking and storing sequential photographs. To assess the evolution of articular lesions, these observations (and hence the arthroscopy) would have to be repeated at least two or three times before any meaningful progress could be appraised. As diagnostic arthroscopy is usually most easily, but not mandatorily, carried out under general anaesthesia and high-thigh tourniquet, severe problems become evident in planning any such study.

LOGISTICS OF USING ARTHROSCOPY

Among surgeons using arthroscopy, the clinical demand for the technique is great. To assess accurately the sequential progress of articular lesions would certainly require a skilled and very experienced operator. However, the ethics of carrying out a minor surgical procedure, albeit one with minimal morbidity, several times on each of a large number of patients are questionable. Arthroscopy can nevertheless be carried out under local anaesthesia (Wredmark and Lundh, 1982), although this makes it more difficult for patient and surgeon alike.

To obtain an observable trend in the prevention of OA with treatment, large numbers of patients would have to be involved. Jackson (1968) showed in a radiological study that five years after a meniscectomy 27% of the knees showed evidence of OA compared with 5% in the control, opposite knee. Jayson (personal communication) has calculated that, to demonstrate a statistically significant reduction from 27% to 15% by giving meniscectomy subjects preventive therapy for five years, 825 patients would need to be entered into such a study. To base such a study on arthroscopy would be unthinkable, particularly at a time in the nation's health when it is difficult enough to find an arthroscope, an operating theatre and a bed from which to accomplish a spectacularly successful operation. I therefore suggest that Jayson's excellent proposition should be directed to radiological assessment of patients after meniscectomy.

MUST THE ARTICULAR CARTILAGE BE STUDIED TO MEASURE THE PROGRESS OF OA?

Noble *et al.* (1980) have shown a consistent relationship between the thickness and structure of articular cartilage, the meniscus and the subchondral bone beneath them. Thus computerised tomography, xero-radiography or even conventional tomography to a fixed reference point may be an advance on the methods available to Jackson (1968).

Waxman and Sledge (1973) have shown a relationship between the clinical status of an arthritic condition and the activity of lysosomal enzymes from the same synovium. Read and co-workers (1982) have demonstrated in an *in vitro* tissue-culture model that synovia from a wide variety of joint afflictions will degrade viable bovine nasal cartilage substrate. The degree of proteoglycan release from that substrate appeared to mirror the severity of the joint affliction. There may thus be some attraction in studying synovial activity as an indicator of cartilage degeneration, or even the threat of it.

Returning finally to arthroscopy, it has to be stressed that the frequency and ubiquity of articular pathology in the adult knee, as outlined at the outset of this article, pose the question as to how valuable arthroscopic observations may be, however skilfully and accurately they are made. Comparing findings from successive examinations would be as difficult as revisiting the same wood five years consecutively and observing the extent of the autumn tints, in an attempt to measure the speed of onset of winter.

MENISCECTOMY CASES AS AN EXPERIMENTAL MODEL

Jayson (personal communication) emphasises the potential of patients who have suffered a meniscectomy to act as 'experimental animals' for the study of influences upon the onset and progression of OA. The literature (Fairbank, 1948; Gear, 1967; Huckell, 1965; Tapper and Hoover, 1969) is replete with references to the fact that meniscectomy is not a benign procedure. However, it must be emphasised here that the term 'meniscectomy' is applied to a variety of operative procedures:

    i. total meniscectomy—by open arthrotomy
    ii. subtotal meniscectomy—by open arthrotomy
    iii. partial meniscectomy—by open arthrotomy
    iv. subtotal meniscectomy—by arthroscopy
    v. partial meniscectomy—by arthroscopy

Jackson (1976) has reported that in a prospective trial in which he compared total meniscectomy with partial meniscectomy, by open arthrotomy, the early results were so much better in the partial meniscectomy cases that he deemed it almost unethical to continue with the study. Now that partial meniscectomy can

be achieved so readily by arthroscopic means the difference between the techniques is sure to be even more striking.

In my view total meniscectomy, in any case other than irreparable peripheral separation of the meniscus, is quite indefensible. Seedhom *et al.* (1979) have elegantly shown that the meniscus functions by absorbing stress as a hoop. Any break in that circle thus disrupts the dissipation of hoop stresses. It is for that reason that Noble *et al.* (1982) have been able to show that residual rims (or rings) of only part of the meniscus can still function as a hoop and thus are worthy of preservation at knee surgery. These points are made to stress why any studies using meniscectomy cases must itemise and standardise the meaning and extent of the 'meniscectomy' used.

The debate cannot rest there. The entire literature on meniscectomy before the era of arthroscopy was devalued by the frequent failure of authors to classify the lesions which they encountered. In a review of this subject Noble (1980) pointed out that there were a number of authors who did not admit to having removed normal meniscus, whereas the incidence of doing so might in fact be as high as 32%. In the same literature review the reported incidence of bucket-handle tears varied between 0 and 62% and the variance of degenerative horizontal cleavage lesions was 0 to 52%. At the same time Noble (1980) has reviewed the literature on the aetiology and pathology of meniscal tears, and Noble and Abernethy (1979) have also indicated the many different types of meniscal tear. Differences are likely between any underlying histopathology (or lack of it); if, for example, we compare a horizontal cleavage lesion in a 40-year-old with an acute bucket-handle tear in a 20-year-old, then we are comparing two very dissimilar disease processes (Noble, 1975, 1977).

CONCLUSIONS

1. Arthroscopy is the best technique currently available with which to study accurately the status of all intra-articular structures.

2. To undertake this procedure in a large number of people, several times each, would be ethically dubious and quite impractical in the current British National Health Service.

3. Arthroscopic observations would have to be interpreted in the light of the knowledge that intra-articular degeneration and other lesions are extremely common and random once skeletal maturity has been achieved.

4. Arthroscopy can be used to operate surgically within the knee. Synovial biopsy specimens can very readily be obtained in this way. It may be relevant to study synovium, as well as articular cartilage, in the measurement of degenerative joint disease.

5. The human being subjected to meniscectomy is highlighted as an excellent 'animal model' for the study of OA, but students of this condition must accurately standardise the description of

the meniscectomy technique used and the nature of the tear thus treated.

6. Medicine is generally concerned with keeping its customers happy. Thus, ultimately, the best way of monitoring a painful condition must be to measure pain and patient contentment.

REFERENCES

BEITZKE, H. (1912) Über die sogenannte Arthritis Deformans Atrophica. *Klin. Med.* **74**, 215–229.

BENNETT, G.A., WAINE, J. and BAUER, W. (1942) *Changes in the Knee Joint at Various Ages.* The Commonwealth Fund, New York.

DANDY, D.J. (1981) *Arthroscopic Surgery of the Knee.* Churchill Livingstone, Edinburgh.

DANDY, D.J. and JACKSON, R.W. (1975) The impact of arthroscopy on the management of disorders of the knee. *J. Bone Joint Surg.* **57**B, 346–348.

DE HAVEN, K.E. and COLLINS, H.R. (1975) Diagnosis of internal derangements of the knee. *J. Bone Joint Surg.* **57**B, 802.

FAHMY, N.R.M., NOBLE, J. and WILLIAMS, E.A. (1981) Relationship betwen meniscal tears and osteoarthritis of the knee. *J. Bone Joint Surg.* **63**B, 653–629.

FAIRBANK, T.J. (1948) Knee joint changes after meniscectomy. *J. Bone Joint Surg.* **30**B, 664–670.

GEAR, M.W.L. (1967) The late results of meniscectomy. *Br. J. Surg.* **54**, 270–272.

HUCKELL, J.R. (1965) Is meniscectomy a benign procedure? *Can. J. Surg.* **8**, 254–260.

IRELAND, J., TRICKEY, E.L. and STOKER, D.J. (1980) Arthroscopy and arthrography of the knee: a critical review. *J. Bone Joint Surg.* **62**B, 3–6.

JACKSON, J.P. (1968) Degenerative changes in the knee after meniscectomy. *Br. Med. J.* **2**, 525–527.

JACKSON, R.W. (1976) Results of partial and total meniscectomy. Presentation to A.A.O.S. Course on Arthroscopy, Boston, USA.

NOBLE, J., DAVIES, D.R.A., MALMISON, P.D., WILLIAMS, E.A., CARDEN, D.G. and STEINGOLD, R.F. (1984) Arthrotomy and meniscectomy: day case procedures. *J. R. Coll. Surg. Edinb.* **29**, 172–175.

NOBLE, J. (1975) Clinical features of the degenerate meniscus with results of meniscectomy. *Br. J. Surg.* **62**, 977–981.

NOBLE, J. (1976) Demonstration to Combined Meeting English Speaking Orthopaedic Associations, Edinburgh.

NOBLE, J. (1977) Lesions of the meniscus. Autopsy incidence in adults less than 55 years old. *J. Bone Joint Surg.* **59**A, 480–483.

NOBLE, J. (1980) Ch.M. Thesis *In Defence of the Meniscus.* University of Edinburgh.

NOBLE, J. and ABERNETHY, P.J. (1979) The painful knee. *Br. J. Hosp. Med.* **14**, 169–171.

NOBLE, J. and ERAT, K. (1980) In defence of the meniscus. A prospective study of 200 meniscectomy patients. *J. Bone Joint Surg.* **62**B, 7–11.

NOBLE, J. and HAMBLEN, D.L. (1975) The pathology of the degenerate meniscus lesions. *J. Bone Joint Surg.* **57**B, 180–186.

NOBLE, J., FAWELL, J.K., HALL, E.P. and SMITH, E. (1980) The relationship of tibial subchondral bone density to the meniscus and to articular fibrillation. *J. Bone Joint Surg.* **62**B, 254.

NOBLE, J., DIAMOND, R., WALKER, G. and SYKES, H. (1982) The functional capacity of disordered menisci. *J. R. Coll. Surg. Edinb.* **27**, 13–20.

READ, L., NOBLE, J., ALEXANDER, K. and COLLINS, R.F. (1982) The action of diseased synovium on cartilage substrate. *J. Bone Joint Surg.* **64**B, 383–384.

SEEDHOM, B.B., DOWSON, D. and WRIGHT, V. (1979) On the 'bucket handle' tear: Partial or total meniscectomy. *J. Bone Joint Surg.* **61**B, 535.

SMILLIE, I.S. (1980) *Diseases of the Knee Joint.* Churchill Livingstone, Edinburgh.

TAPPER, E.M. and HOOVER, N.W. (1969) Late results after meniscectomy. *J. Bone Joint Surg.* **51**A, 517–526.

WAXMAN, B. and SLEDGE, C.B. (1973) Correlation of histochemical, histologic and biochemical evaluations of human synovium with clinical activity. *Arthritis Rheum.* **16**, 376–383.

WREDMARK, T. and LUNDH, R. (1982) Arthroscopy under local anaesthesia using controlled pressure-irrigation with prilocaine. *J. Bone Joint Surg.* **64**B, 583–585.

Chapter 13

Scope of Radiology

I. WATT

Department of Radiodiagnosis, Bristol Royal Infirmary, Bristol, UK

Most OA changes observed radiologically are qualitative and hard to quantify. Standard measurements of joint-space width are, however, available for normal hips (Fredensborg and Nisson, 1978), and knees (Hall and Wyshak, 1980). While changes in these may be assessed from plain film images, meticulous attention to detail is necessary to obtain reproducible results. Many factors can introduce error, particularly magnification, which may produce a 25–40% artefact (Hall and Wyshak, 1980), but also obliquity and the absence of specific end-points or landmarks in most joints. Without opacification of the joint surfaces it is not possible to tell what occupies the radiolucent gap between bony cortices — hyaline cartilage, joint fluid or pannus — or whether the hyaline cartilage itself is uniform in thickness. Moreover, knee arthrography has revealed differences in joint space between the medial and lateral compartments and between sexes (Hall and Wyshak, 1980). To detect the full extent of joint-space narrowing in large joints it may be necessary to obtain weight-bearing films, but the joint space may then appear to be widened in one part and narrowed in another, hindering assessment of hyaline cartilage loss (Leach *et al.*, 1970); varus and valgus stress films may however be helpful in determining the true joint space.

Computerised tomography is unlikely to provide precise measurements because of the difficulties in establishing endpoints and obtaining images normal to joint surfaces.

There is a marked variation in joint morphology with age, joint-space width and swelling being age- as well as sex-dependent (Mäkelä *et al.*, 1979). Comparisons between individuals or with a normal population may therefore not be meaningful. Some forms of arthritis, e.g. gout and multicentric reticulohystiocystosis, are characterised by apparent preservation of joint-space width until late in the disease process. In certain conditions, such as acromegaly or cretinism, there is a true increase in hyaline-cartilage thickness, and an apparent increase is observed in Perthes' disease. In such circumstances, the assessment of joint-space narrowing is clearly more complex than in control populations.

The appearances in common conditions such as osteoarthritis and rheumatoid disease show great variation, making comparisons between individuals suspect, particularly in small series. A frank deterioration in joint morphology may even be associated with an apparent increase in joint-space width in, for example, a Charcot joint. Finally, it is important to consider the time scale against which joint-space narrowing or restitution is being judged; the early increase in joint-space width observed following hip osteotomy for osteoarthritis appears to be transient, for instance, to judge by appearances at five years (Weisl, 1980).

Bone scanning (scintigraphy) provides the single most sensitive means of assessing degenerative arthritis at the knee, compared with clinical examination, radiography (with and without weight-bearing) and double-contrast arthrography (Thomas *et al.*, 1975). The data obtained can be interpreted in two main ways. First, increased activity in the joint during the early bloodpool phase of the bone scan correlates with joint tenderness and inflammation. Second, increased activity in the delayed image seems to correspond to active bone formation. A positive improvement in the scintigraphic features of a diseased joint may therefore be more informative than the continued preservation, or even apparent improvement, of radiographic joint space width. Compared with radiographic appearances, which take at least two weeks to develop, scintigraphy reflects activity at the time of injection, which may be an important consideration in crossover drug trials. However, quantitation from a skeletal scintigram is also fraught with difficulty, and a visual scoring system may be both easier to employ and more objective.

REFERENCES

Fredensborg, N. and Nisson, B.E. (1978) The joint space in normal hip radiographs. *Radiology* **126**, 325–326.

Hall, F.M. and Wyshak, G. (1980) Thickness of articular cartilage in the normal knee. *J. Bone Joint Surg.* **62**A, 408–413.

Leach, R.E., Gregg, T. and Siber, F.J. (1970) Weight bearing radiography in osteoarthritis of the knee. *Radiology* **97**, 265–268.

Mäkelä, P., Virtama, P. and Dean, P.B. (1979) Finger joint swelling; correlation with age, gender and manual labor. *Am. J. Roentgenol.* A**132**, 939–943.

Thomas, T.H., Resnick, D., Alazraki, N., Daniel, D. and Greenfield, R. (1975) Compartmental evaluation of osteoarthritis of the knee. *Radiology* **116**, 585–594.

Weisl, H. (1960) Intertrochanteric osteotomy for osteoarthritis. *J. Bone Joint Surg.* **62**B, 37–42.

Chapter 14

Scope of Radioisotope Measurements

D. M. GRENNAN

University of Manchester Rheumatic Diseases Centre, Hope Hospital, Manchester, UK

The problems of assessing OA in man include definition of normality in the population to be studied and the difficulty of obtaining age-matched controls, definition of the phases of the disease and its distinction from the slow progression of 'naturally-occurring' age-related changes. Patients who present clinically with OA are almost certainly being studied during the late and symptomatic phase of their illness when the primary arthritic disease process, whatever that is due to, has become complicated by secondary processes including inflammation and attempts at repair. The early phase of the disease, which is more likely to be amenable to preventive drug treatment, may be asymptomatic. Features of OA which assessment techniques should attempt to measure include *symptoms* such as pain, stiffness and loss of function, together with the inflammatory element, both of which probably develop late in the disease process, and the *basic features* of bone hypertrophy and cartilage loss.

Available isotope techniques include counting or imaging after intravenous injection of sodium pertechnetate (^{99m}Tc) or of ^{99m}Tc-labelled diphosphonates or pyrophosphate. The first of these methods, ^{99m}Tc imaging, probably detects mainly the inflammatory aspects of peripheral joint disease. By contrast, ^{99m}Tc methylene diphosphonate or pyrophosphate are both bone-seeking isotopes, more likely to be of use in the assessment of bone hypertrophy and osteophytosis. Cartilage metabolism, although it may be measured in experimental animals by the uptake of tritiated glucosamine or other compounds, cannot be measured clinically in man as no suitable gamma-emitting isotope is available.

Whole body retention studies with bone-seeking isotopes have been used to demonstrate the generalised increase of bone turnover in rheumatoid arthritis. It seems unlikely that such a technique would be of much practical value in OA. However, local imaging with ^{99m}Tc methylene diphosphonate can demonstrate OA changes both in peripheral joints and in the spine. These techniques still present some unresolved problems, notably quantification of peripheral joint uptake and definition of the optimum time to scan following intravenous injection of the isotope. It also remains to ascertain whether isotope scanning really detects early actively-progressing disease, rather than established changes, and to determine the sensitivity of the technique for the detection of early OA, as compared to clinical and radiological measurements. These questions could be studied in an animal model of OA.

Index